THE
ATHLETE'S
CLOCK

CONTENTS

FOREWORD

Once upon a time the understanding of exercise physiology was easy. The key to all forms of exercise performance was the heart, whose function determined how far and how fast humans can run, swim, or cycle. Once the heart's limiting capacity is reached, the muscles become oxygen deficient, releasing poisonous lactic acid. The lactic acid interferes with normal muscle function, causing the anguish we recognize as fatigue. According to this explanation, the best athletes are those with the largest hearts, best able to pump the most blood to their active muscles and produce the highest rates of oxygen consumption during exercise.

It is a theory based on work done by the British Nobel Laureates Sir Frederick Gowland Hopkins in 1907 and Professor Archibald Vivian Hill in the 1920s. This idea has been widely promoted and vigorously defended by legions of exercise scientists ever since. Most humans with any interest in exercise science believe this theory to be the only possible truth.

But for the first time in 90 years, the past decade has witnessed the appearance of some cracks in the walls of this fortress of belief. We now know that some things are not easily explained by this traditional Hopkins-Hill model. If the model is the final truth, then there really is no need for athletic competitions. Medals can simply be given to those with the largest hearts and the greatest capacity to consume oxygen. But the problem is that the very best distance runners (the Kenyans and Ethiopians, for example) do not have any greater capacity to consume oxygen than do lesser runners who finish far, far behind. Thus something other than simply a big heart and a large capacity to consume oxygen must explain truly exceptional athletic performance.

Indeed, this theory invites the simplest question: If the heart limits all forms of endurance exercise performance, why do cyclists in the Tour de France or runners in the Olympic marathon race at submaximal levels of heart function? If the heart is indeed the factor limiting their performances, then those athletes' hearts must begin to function at maximal effort the instant the race begins. But their hearts do not. Hence, something else is involved.

Probably the most damning evidence against this traditional theory is the simplest and most obvious—so obvious, in fact, that it has been ignored for the past 90 years: Can the Hopkins-Hill model explain how athletes pace themselves not just during races but also during training?

If the control of exercise performance resides in the exercising muscles under the action of this toxic lactic acid, then why do athletes begin races of different distances at different paces? If lactic acid is the sole determinant of an athlete's pace, then there can be only one exercise pace for each individual regardless of the distance she plans to cover. The pace must be that at which the effect of the poisonous lactic acid is just being felt. Going any faster will cause more lactic acid to be produced, slowing the performance. But slowing down will cause a drop in lactic acid levels in the muscles, removing its inhibitory effect and leading to an immediate (but temporary) increase in performance. Soon, however, the higher intensity will lead to increased lactic acid production in the muscles, reversing the process.

If the model is completely unable to clarify how different paces are possible during exercise, it has even greater difficulty explaining what happens near the end of the exercise as athletes begin to speed up in anticipation of the finish—the classic end spurt. The end spurt is most obvious at the finish of each stage of the Tour de France but is present in all running races longer than 800 meters. How is it possible for an exhausted athlete to speed up at the end of a race when he is the most fatigued? This common phenomenon indicates that our understanding of fatigue—classically defined in all textbooks of exercise physiology as the inability to sustain the desired muscle force (or running speed)—is utterly incapable of explaining what happens in the real world of competitive sport. If athletes speed up at the end of races when they should be the most tired, they cannot be fatigued, according to this hallowed physiological definition.

And even more confusing is this: As they sprint for the line in the final moments of their end spurts, athletes do not activate all the available muscle fibers in their exercising limbs. They always finish with muscular reserve. Which raises these questions: Why not? What is holding them back? And even more intriguing is this: If an athlete finishes second, milliseconds behind the first athlete, what was holding her back? Why did she not risk death by exercising just a little harder in order to win the race? The conclusion must be that she chose to come in second rather than to go faster even if going faster would not have killed her.

Then the final piece of evidence against this purely peripheral control of exercise performance is that certain substances can have a marked effect on human exercise performance even though they act only on the brain. The most obvious example is amphetamines, a class of drugs that dramatically improve performance by acting on the brain to reduce the uncomfortable sensations of fatigue.

In the face of such compelling evidence, one could expect that supporters of this traditional explanation would acknowledge that their model might not be absolutely correct. Science is supposed to be a courteous activity conducted by decorous men and women according to time-honored principles of fair play and respect for differing opinions, all for a singular goal: the pursuit of a perfect truth. Sadly, the reality is sometimes different. Modern science, and perhaps even more so in exercise science, is a war waged on opposing sides by men and women with varying measures of self-importance. Those most certain of their opinions are usually also the most belligerent.

Those intrepid nonbelievers who question soon attract the scorn of the majority. The result is that it is much easier to stay quiet or to choose conformity. It is into this hostile arena that the genial Dr. Thomas Rowland and his sagacious book have made their entry.

Dr. Rowland, a pediatric cardiologist, is lean and athletic—a lifetime athlete. His small, linear frame identifies him as an ectomorph. According to 1940s Harvard psychologist William Sheldon, the defining characteristic of the ectomorph is cerebrotonia—a greater capacity for deep thinking than for urgent acting. Shakespeare understood that their need to think and to understand more deeply places the ectomorph on the social edge. Of Cassius who plotted his assassination, Julius Caesar is allowed to observe this:

> Yond Cassius has a lean and hungry look,
> He thinks too much; such men are dangerous.

Much better to surround oneself with the soft bellied:

> Let me have men about me that are fat,
> Sleek-headed men and such as sleep a-nights.

In *The Athlete's Clock*, Rowland plots the assassination not of an autocratic emperor. Instead, he invites us to question some of our most hallowed concepts of human athleticism. He wishes to understand how research in sport science helps us better understand how time, aging, our internal biological clocks, and associated controls like the central pattern generator (CPG) influence human athletic performance.

His overarching questions are these: Is the control of physical effort over time—sporting performance—under the conscious control of the athlete? Or do subconscious controls of which we have little knowledge really determine how well we can perform in sport? Thus he poses this question: Are the forces of destiny—or the finish time in a 10K road race—under our conscious control?

Rowland begins by providing evidence from laboratory studies showing that the pacing strategy during more prolonged endurance exercise may be regulated by subconscious controls that produce the uncomfortable symptoms that we recognize as fatigue. He wonders whether these sensations arise "from the unconscious portions of the brain, which, having sensed physiological information indicating high-exercise stress, depress force of muscle contraction and block the desire to continue, all in the name of preserving safety?" He acknowledges that few exercise scientists and even fewer athletes are impressed by any explanation that proposes that human athletes are not in exclusive control of their own sporting performances. In answer, he provides a body of current evidence that allows readers to arrive at a more informed opinion.

The function of those controls is to regulate the frequency and power of the muscle contractions, expressed in running as stride frequency and stride length. Runners achieve this by acting on a CPG that sets the stride frequency and stride length and hence the pace. This simple explanation is revolutionary. Defenders of the Hopkins-Hill model speak not in terms of how a CPG might regulate exercise performance but exclusively in terms of how the heart's nutrient supply to the exercising muscles regulates their function and therefore establishes the runner's pace.

Not that this CPG is a novel evolutionary development unique to athletic humans. Instead, a similar controller subtends the identical function in the more primitive brains of the most ancient creatures like the lowly cockroach. The magic of this CPG is that it will always choose the most efficient combination of contraction frequency and contraction power regardless of the activity—running, swimming, or cycling—and the conditions of exercise. The CPG does its work without requiring any input from conscious thought, although there may be some limited capacity for conscious choice to influence the actions of the CPG in the short term.

What of sprinting speed? Could the peak rate of firing of the (subconscious) CPG determine how fast humans can sprint over 100 meters? Probably not that simple, since this excludes the role of the sprinter's muscles in producing the force necessary to propel the body between strides. Weak muscles and a superfast CPG will still produce a slow 100-meter time. But like distance runners, even 100-meter sprinters must pace themselves. According to Caribbean sprinter Steven Headley in an interview with Rowland, "You can't run all out for more than about 4 or 5 seconds. . . . I really don't know what causes me to slow at the finish. Sometimes I'm not even aware of it." Is this another example of the subconscious control of human athletic performance?

Clear evidence for well-defined subconscious controls is provided by the diurnal (24-hour) variations in human athletic performance. Even better examples are the responses of players in fast ball sports like baseball, tennis, and cricket, in which the ball must be struck on the basis of advanced cues occurring in the very earliest portion of its flight and in which conscious actions can play no part. In all these sports, the ball striker must hit the ball at a time when he does not know the ball's precise position in space (since he does not see it). Nor does he know precisely when the ball will reach the point at which he wishes to strike it. The marvel is that few humans are ever able to make these seemingly improbable actions successfully, let alone most of the time.

Thomas Rowland has written a magical book that is both timely and revolutionary. My wish is that it will open minds to a new possibility: that we know much less about the factors that regulate human athletic performance than in our simple ignorance we may believe. That is the hidden message of this rebellious, indeed heretical, book. It is a message that exercise scientists need to take seriously if we are to advance our profession as a solemn science that aims to detect, rather than to conceal, truth.

Tim Noakes, OMS, MD, DSc
Discovery Health Professor of Exercise and Sports Science,
University of Cape Town and Sports Science Institute
of South Africa

INTRODUCTION

We are all time travelers, passengers on an unflagging moving present that carries us even further into the future.

—Michael Lockwood, The Labyrinth of Time, 2005

Hey, kids! What time is it?

—Buffalo Bob, The Howdy Doody Show, circa 1952

By now it was almost four o'clock, and I was not greatly surprised that he was late.

I was awaiting, with no little anticipation, the visit of an old boyhood friend whom I hadn't seen in decades. It was so long ago, in fact, that it struck me that instead of coming from Michigan, it was more like he would be arriving from a different time dimension altogether. John had been a fairly straight-and-narrow fellow in high school, but after graduation, his life had taken a rather bizarre and certainly unexpected turn. Maybe it was his participation in the 1968 Chicago riots that led John to suddenly drop out of society, moving into a barn in the Lower Peninsula and abandoning a promising future in law, family, and all the usual social conventions. And there he had been ever since.

I had heard enough of his story to expect some rather eccentric behavior. He would, for example, insist on sleeping outdoors (so as, in his words, "not to lose the magic"). But what I did not anticipate was that immediately on his arrival, this bearded, altogether cheerful soul would rapidly stride from room to room, covering up all the clocks with a towel or cloth. We were, it seemed, about to spend the weekend unaware of time. (His idea was not original. The 18th-century philosopher Jean-Jacques Rousseau, in a gesture of disdain for the constraints of time, is said to have tossed away his watch, predating Peter Fonda in the opening scene of *Easy Rider* by a couple of centuries. In Rousseau's case, it is tempting to suggest that this act might have been associated with his subsequent bizarre social behavior, progressive paranoia, and ultimate death with insanity.)

My mind recoiled. How would we know when to eat dinner? To go to bed? When would we know when the coffee shop was opening for my morning latte? We wouldn't know how long to cook the lasagna. Or when to meet our friends at the cinema. And—now seemingly of critical importance—when would John know it was time to leave?

For three days, I was off kilter, disoriented, confused. No question about it, this weekend had a lesson. Those of us who have stuck to the narrow path of a conventional life are slaves to time. Without its anchor, our daily lives are set adrift. (Adventuresome readers are invited to try this experiment for themselves. See what it's like to miss your daughter's piano recital, to burn a steak or two.)

Meaning of Time

Time is, quite literally, of the essence. Indeed, it creates the very boundaries of our lives on this planet. From the moment of our birth, the sand begins to flow without ceasing through the hourglass to mark the point of our exit. In between times, we mark time in all that we do—our sleeping, eating, working, vacations. Clearly, no other single factor so defines our existence.

No wonder, then, that the great thinkers—philosophers, mathematicians, poets, theologians, physicists—have struggled throughout history to understand the nature of time. Time is something we all know about. But what is it?

Aristotle was among the first to consider time as a fundamental feature of the universe. From this viewpoint, it proceeds linearly and continuously, without interruption or influence by outside events. It doesn't matter what you're doing—time marches on. It is like a geometric straight line. Here, likening time to a mathematical construct would reveal its absolute, or physical, nature.

This was a popular idea, since it obviously reflected what people saw before them—the regularity of the tides, seasons, migration of birds, and, most particularly, the progression of the sun, moon, and stars across the sky. This concept of time as an imperturbable progression was further embodied by the invention of the clock, which defined time in respect to astronomical events. This modern measurement of time has, of course, become extraordinarily precise, extending from highly exact astronomical observations to the frequency of vibration of the cesium atom, a clock with an accuracy of 5 parts per 10 million million. That's a margin of error of .0000001 seconds per day.

Others have been inclined to view the passage of time from the standpoint of human experience (*psychological* or *subjective* time). Human beings, among all the animals, are uniquely gifted with the ability to sense time. This is nowhere less apparent than when you are awaiting a flight delayed for three hours (we might call this *O'Hare time*). Subjective time can, of course, move much more rapidly, like when you are enjoying a party with good friends or winning at tennis (label this as *40-love time*). You'd have difficulty convincing yourself that the agonizing creep of time at the airport is identical to that on the tennis court. But viewed from the U.S. Naval observatory in Washington, D.C., the keeper of astronomical time, no objective difference exists between O'Hare and 40-love time.

Time can also be viewed from the perspective of sequence. Gottfried Leibniz (who lived from 1646 to 1716) thought of time that way. (He also invented calculus, the binary system on which today's computers are based, and—to his lasting credit—optimism in life.) According to this idea, termed the *relational theory of time*, events do not take place in time; instead, it's the other way around. Time is defined by the order in which events occur. By this concept, events in life become the cornerstone of existence rather than time itself. This argument runs counter to that of time as a physical, immutable, independent reality.

You could easily fill an entire library with what's been written about the nature of time. (Those who wish a concise, easily readable source can try the 1972 book *What is Time?* by the British author G.J. Whitrow from Oxford Press.) Among these discourses are many intriguing themes. For instance, Einstein's ideas on relativity spoke against time as an absolute, stating that the passage of time depends on the location and speed of the person looking at the clock. In effect, a clock traveling at extraordinary speeds will appear to slow down when compared to another clock at rest relative to the observer. Such arguments are inconsistent with a physical, independent characterization of time. They state that rather than being absolute and invariable, time is related to speed. Thus, they are more supportive of Leibniz's concept of relative time. (Until your Volvo can approach the speed of light, however, these can be considered theoretical, rather than pragmatic, arguments.)

And then there is the question of the arrow of time. Can time go backwards? Or is it unidirectional? In light of our daily experiences, this would seem a bit silly. Of course, billiard balls do not come flying out of their corner pockets, your mother-in-law's precious china dish that you dropped cannot suddenly reassemble itself, the faux pas you uttered at the boss' dinner party last night cannot be retrieved.

Others have not been so sure. Physical laws of motion, for example, work just as well in reverse as they do in forward motion. That is, if you filmed a system corresponding to the laws of Newtonian mechanics, you would never be able to tell whether the film was later being projected backward or forward. It is possible to calculate not only the future positions of the planets around the solar system, but also their locations in the past. In the laws of physics, there is no preferred direction of physical processes in respect to time.

Indeed, this question of the direction of time has been considered with a great deal of thoughtful deliberation, and a number of books have been devoted entirely to this subject alone.[1] In the end, it seems that common expectation holds true. Students of the subject have generally come to the conclusion that the passage of time, notwithstanding events in certain popular novels and films, cannot be put in reverse. It proceeds only forward. The most powerful argument for one direction of time comes from the second law of thermodynamics, which holds that the degree of disorder, or *entropy*, in a system increases as a function of time. Left to themselves, systems become more disorganized, not the reverse. Predictably, things run down. Other evidence of the one-way arrow of time has been witnessed in the course of biological evolution, the chronological order of geological events, and the extended trends of astronomical events (like the life spans of stars or the expansion of the universe itself).

Another interesting perspective of time is that in its linear progressive flow, there exists no such thing as *now*. Like its counterpart in mathematics, the point representing the present is dimensionless. It, in fact, does not exist. As soon as you consider the point of now as the present, it has become part of the past. Contrary to all you learned about Zen theory, not to mention *carpe diem*, by this account, you cannot live for the present because the present does not exist. There is only future and past. As Kai Krause has concluded, "Everything is about the anticipation of the moment and the memory of the moment, but not the moment."

The only way to make time stand still, as it were, is to think about it in terms of duration between two points in immediate time. That is, "I am now a student at the University of New Mexico." In this way, now becomes a state, a condition. And you could, I guess, remain a perpetual college student, thereby freezing time indefinitely.

And, finally, being linked so intimately with the essence of human existence, it comes as no surprise that poets and philosophers have waxed nostalgic on just how precious time is. Consider this quote from Fernando Pessoa:

> I sorely grieve over time's passage. It's always with exaggerated emotion that I leave something behind, whatever it may be. The miserable rented room where I lived for a few months, the dinner table at the provincial hotel where I stayed for six days, even the sad waiting room at the station where I spent two hours waiting for a train—yes, their loss grieves me. But the special things in life—when I leave them behind and realize with all my nerves' sensibility that I'll never see or have them again, at least not in that exact same moment—grieve me metaphysically. A chasm opens up in my soul and a cold breeze of the hour of God blows across my pallid face.[2]

Chronological Versus Physiological Time

In 1884, a group of international astronomers gathered in Washington, DC, to create worldwide time zones. Their goal: to eliminate the chaos and confusion that had previously existed as each locality in the world sought to create its own particular time measure. In the United States, for instance, each railroad company set train arrivals and departures by its own time standard. The year before this historic meeting, almost 100 different railroad times were in force.

The world was divided into 24 longitudinal time zones to put us all in synch. They chose Greenwich, England, on the outskirts of London, as the starting point, or the *prime meridian*. (Today on visiting this site, one expects to see something extraordinary, maybe a bright yellow line running north and south through the grounds, but, no.) What was formalized in the capital city of the United States was the original idea of the ancient Babylonians a couple of thousand centuries earlier. This was to divide the day into 24 hours, with 60 minutes to an hour, and 60 seconds to a minute. This is all related, of course, to astronomical events, which define the chronological time that governs our lives.

Biological activities all vary rhythmically, in a manner that roughly approximates chronological time as well. Body temperature, heart rate, and blood pressure all wax and wane over specific time periods. Some of these *circadian rhythms* have direct bearing on sports performance. Chapter 4 deals with this phenomenon in more depth.

Another way that biological functions relate to the passage of time is the rate over time at which physiological processes take place. Scientists, in their attempts to define the real world as we see it, are accustomed to examining biological structure and function in concrete, three-dimensional terms, measuring things in grams, meters, or liters. However, recognition is growing that time, that impalpable factor of the fourth dimension, plays a critical role in how biological systems function. Most specifically, it is clear that such function must be couched in terms of its duration, or how long it takes to occur.

Functional activities of the body, such as sweating, cellular metabolism, or the rate of blood filtered by the kidney in the production of urine, all occur at a certain level of intensity related to time. Using these same examples, then, we can talk about the number of milliliters of sweat produced in a minute, or metabolic rate in terms of the oxygen used by cells as liters per minute, or urine production in milliliters per hour. In the same way, we can also talk about time defining broader biological processes, such as life span or generation time (time between conception and the age of ability to procreate). We can define the limits of such functions, compare them between different people, and define abnormal functions (as in diseased conditions), all by describing their activities in respect to the time it takes for them to occur.

No surprises yet. But here's the interesting thing. The rates of these functions are not associated with chronological time at all. Somehow they missed the memo from Greenwich. Instead, intriguingly, they relate to body weight, or *mass*. The bigger you are, the slower these processes go in respect to chronological, or clock time, and the longer it takes them (on your watch) to occur. The heart rate per minute of a shrew, which weighs about 2.5 grams, is about 1,000 times in a minute. During the same time period, the heart of an elephant beats only 30 times, and a human being's beats 70 times.

The same thing is true of rate of energy turnover within a mammal's cells when metabolism is expressed relative to the animal's size. That is, the smaller an animal, the more intensely its metabolic fires burn. The daily energy metabolism of a 30-gram mouse approximates 170 kilocalories for each kilogram of its body mass. A 300-kilogram cow uses about one-tenth as much, or 17 kilocalories per kilogram. Everything small animals do happens faster than the actions of big ones. It is not the chronological clock that dictates the speed of physiological function, but rather, body size.[3]

We can express this link between physiological functional time and body mass by a kind of mathematical equation called an *allometric formula*:

$$Y = aM^b$$

Here, Y is a biological process (liters of blood per minute, or times between breaths), M is body mass, a is a proportionality constant, and b (the most important item) is the scaling factor that indicates the extent and direction of the relationship between changes in the variable Y and body mass. A value of 1.0 for b indicates that the rate of the biological function increases in direct proportion to body mass. That would be true for respiratory rate, for example, if an animal weighing 10 kilograms breathed 20 times per minute, while a 40-kilogram animal breathed 80 times per minute. If $b = 0$, body mass would have no relationship to the process Y. Values between zero and 1.0 tell us that the biological process Y is associated with body mass, but Y increases at a faster rate than mass does as an animal's size increases.

What is striking is that when one considers various physiological functions in different groups of animals, there is a rather remarkable frequency of values for the mass scaling exponent b that approximate 0.25. In fact, William Calder was able to find 40 allometric equations in the research literature that related the time duration of different physiological processes in animals with body mass, all of which had a value of b between 0.25 and 0.39. The sidebar illustrates a few examples.

On examining this list, there is another intriguing observation. One cannot help being struck, not only by the consistency of quarter-power scaling exponents (that is, b is about 0.25) on this list, but also by the

Allometric relationships between rate of biological functions and body mass (*M*) of adult mammals (compiled from multiple sources).

Life span, in captivity (years) 11.6 $M^{0.20}$

Reproductive maturity (years) 0.75 $M^{0.29}$

Gestation period (days) 65 $M^{0.25}$

Erythrocyte life span (days) 23 $M^{0.18}$

Plasma albumin half life (days) 5 $M^{0.32}$

Glomerular filtration rate (min.) 6.5 $M^{0.27}$

Blood circulation time (sec.) 21 $M^{0.21}$

Respiratory cycle (sec.) 1.1 $M^{0.26}$

Cardiac cycle (sec.) 0.25 $M^{0.25}$

Metabolic rate per kg (min.) 70 $M^{-0.25}$

wide diversity of the biological functions included. Indeed, at least at first blush, they seem to have no obvious mechanistic connection at all. By what link could one assume, for example, that the rate of urine filtration in the kidney has any commonality with the twitch contraction of the soleus muscle? How about time to reproductive maturity in respect to the relationship to how much one weighs? What do these functions have in common that would give them nearly identical associations with body mass?

Even the duration of life itself fits into this scheme, with a mass exponent of 0.20. From this observation, Calder remarked that "using maximum life span, rather than absolute time, it appears that each life comprises about the same number of physiologic events or actions; in other words, each animal lives its life faster or slower governed by size, but accomplishes just as much biologically, whether large or small."[3]

It's almost as if we were born with a certain bank account of physiological function. The faster we use them up (in this analogy, make withdrawals from the account), the shorter our life expectancy. The average mouse has a 3-year life span, with a heart rate of 600 beats per minute (bpm), while the elephant lives 40 years, with a heart rate of 30 bpm. Yet their total number of heartbeats in a life time is similar. (Fortunately for you and me, human beings are outliers in this relationship. If we were to fit the pattern of other mammals, we would use up our allocated total of heartbeats by the time we reached age 25.)

A consideration of the obvious question of just why body mass is linked to the duration of physiological processes and events begs more time and space than is available here. The bottom line is that no one knows for sure. Attempts have been made to explain the mass scaling exponents for individual functions. But the ubiquitousness of quarter-power values for b, even in processes as seemingly far removed as breathing rate, kidney glomerular filtration rate, and generation time, seem to indicate there is a universal underlying principle involved.

Even if you're thrown by the math, the message should be clear. We can't rely on physiological processes to follow chronological time—they march to a different drummer. And that can be important when studying those functions that influence physical fitness and sport performance.

Before leaving this issue of physiological time, another aspect of biological timekeeping relative to sport performance deserves mentioning. The many factors that combine to determine athletic prowess are extraordinarily complex, but they share one feature in common—during the course of childhood development, they progressively evolve, or mature, toward the adult state. These advances in physical, physiological, and psychosocial features are predictably translated into steady improvements in motor performance (whether the child is engaged in sports or not). But, once again, the tempo of biological development is not closely attuned to chronological time. Here, the biological clock is set largely by genetic factors. The rate of this process during the course of the childhood years can vary dramatically among children. Thus, at any given chronological age, you may witness wide differences in body size, composition, physiological function, motor skill, personality, and motivation. As Bob Malina, anthropologist and sport scientist who has written extensively on this subject, has emphasized, "biologic processes have their own timetables and do not celebrate birthdays."[4] It is not difficult to appreciate the potential effect of this issue on early selection of talent, or the matching of competitors in contact sports like football. But this is a big subject. Chapter 6 presents a discussion with Professor Malina in more detail.

Athletes and Time

Athletes, it hardly deserves stating, are no strangers to the importance of time. Sometimes, in fact, time is the very point of the sport. How much time elapses while you run 100 meters as fast as you can? In other sports, time regulates the duration of the competition. How many times can a group of five unusually tall players throw a ball through a round hoop in 40 minutes? Indeed, without a clock, most competitive sports would become quite meaningless. Yet, in other events, such as tennis or baseball, the timing of muscular action largely defines athletic skill.

Athletes are also keenly interested in their repeated performances over time. They become fixated on batting averages, fighting records, or field goal percentages. When repeated performances are unexpectedly poor, we talk about athletes being in a slump. When Michael Jordan sinks six three-pointers in a row in the NBA finals against Portland, he's on a hot streak. What explains these runs? Since the athletes have typically experienced no physical changes at the time, we say they are more (or less) mentally focused. We hear them described as trying too hard or, when on a roll, just letting it flow. Getting hot is something all athletes strive for (and would be willing, no doubt, to give a lot to know the secret of why it was happening).

It comes as a bit of surprise, then, that people who know a lot about the statistics of randomness are quick to pooh-pooh such explanations. Being hot or in a slump, they say, is just a matter of chance.

Thomas Gilovich from Cornell University teamed up with Stanford colleagues Robert Vallone and Amos Tversky to analyze the success of streak shooting of the Philadelphia 76ers professional basketball team during seasons from 1980 to 1982. Their findings? "Variations in shooting percentages across games do not deviate from their overall shooting percentages enough to produce significantly more hot (or cold) nights than expected by chance alone."[5]

What they're saying is that if you flip a coin many, many times, you will eventually witness 10 heads in a row. Not often, but by chance, it will occur. And if you shoot a ball at a basket a large number of times, at some point, you will sink 10 in a row. Neither of you is more mentally focused. You're both in a groove, but only by statistical chance.[5] (What bothers me about this analysis is that it seems that the people who have hot streaks always have names like DiMaggio and Jordan!)

Sometimes, too, athletes take great efforts to slow down time. Witness the interminable bouncing of the ball or tugging at the pants of my favorite pro tennis players (who will remain unnamed here) before they finally serve. Or the Yankees and the Red Sox, berated by

Yogi's Wisdom

These pages would be incomplete without checking in to hear what Yogi Berra, baseball's resident philosopher, had to say about time. In fact, the keen malapropisms made by the former catcher for the New York Yankees contain useful insights about how we should think about this valuable commodity. Here are a few examples:

(When asked the time) "You mean, now?"

"The future ain't what it used to be."

"It gets late early out there."

"It's like déjà vu all over again."

"I usually take a two-hour nap, from one o'clock to four."

And everybody's favorite, "It ain't over until it's over."

(Just to keep things straight, I shouldn't put on airs like I know a lot about Yogi and the Yankees. I once possessed, I think, a Yogi Berra baseball card. I got a view of Yankee Stadium during a Circle Line boat tour around Manhattan when I was nine. And I have a friend who lives in Memphis, Bruce Alpert, who attends Yankees fantasy baseball camps. But that's about it.)

umpires for taking their sweet time. Not to mention golfers on the PGA tour who dawdle on the back nine. The most obvious, though, are the basketball teams in the era before the shot clock who tried to protect their lead by stalling out the final minutes of play (see chapter 3).

Athletes, too, are very conscious of how time is best proportioned as they construct their training schedules. This *periodization*, or pattern of training, appears to influence gains in performance and permits peaking for big events. Athletes need to decide just how many weeks they should use high- and low-intensity training, how many days a week to devote to speed work, how many days of rest they should take, and how many days they should taper before a big competition.

All that training gets funneled down into those small particles of time we call competition. That's what it's all about. Athletes have taken their genetic gifts, done everything in their power to enhance them, and now—in just a few clicks of the clock—they must realize them.

This phenomenon is seen through moments in time that, often in dramatic fashion, serve to define the essence of sports itself. Carlton Fisk willing his drive to left field into fair territory during the sixth game of the 1975 World Series. John Landy glancing over his left shoulder as Roger Bannister passed by him on the outside in the final lap to win the mile of the century in Vancouver. Michael Jordan in full flight above the rim. Here, time is stilled—at least in memories and photographs—and moments are imbued with powerful meaning for the world of competitive sports.

Some have attributed spiritual qualities to such moments. In his 1999 book *The Tao of the Jump Shot* (Seastone Publishers), John Mahoney writes, "Although the jump shot is a dynamic movement of energy, there is one unique point, a nearly measureless instant, during which the athlete remains frozen in space. The point of release, born in a moment of stillness. . ."

Sometimes, rarely, remarkably, athletes seem to transcend the tyranny of time altogether. Like Roger Bannister on the final straightaway: "There was no pain, only a great unity of movement and aim." In the throes of supreme physical effort, they've been transported somewhere else, someplace where even the clock doesn't matter. Victor Price, in his short story "The Other Kingdom," wrote about this:

> As they entered the straight they moved into a purely physical kingdom. Nothing mattered now but to keep going. . . . It was a wave of feral aggression, a lust for power and at the same time a sacred terror, as though he were pursued by some fierce and inescapable beast. Life existed now only as far as the finishing tape. The element of time expanded and contracted simultaneously; a seriousness on the threshold of physical agony, where the

actions of this one man were determining the fate of all men, and none of the rules of life applied anymore. There was no good, no evil, no success, no failure. There was only the man eternally running. . . .[6]

(Alas, for most of us mere mortals, crossing the finishing line of a race is more likely to be accompanied by waves of nausea, hunger for air, cramps, and the longing for a warm shower.)

What's Ahead in This Book

These pages explore ways that considerations of time and its relationship to work effort might optimize sport performance. This is our central theme. From many perspectives, this book shows that the influences of time on sport success are seemingly fixed, outside the athlete's control. Our muscles weaken as we age, we swing a bat in milliseconds at an oncoming fastball, our leg muscles contract in a beautifully synchronized harmony during a 10K road race. All these lie in different levels of time, in which we have little say over the matter.

But this book also poses some interesting and challenging questions about just how much athletes can or should try to manipulate time to their advantage. If physiological responses to training vary rhythmically during the course of a day, would it be rewarding to select these times to head to the track? If a coach thinks that a high stroke count leads to a better time in a particular swimming event, should the athlete go with it? Or is it better to stick to a cadence that feels intuitively more normal—one directed by a subconscious controller of stroke tempo in the brain? Be forewarned that the answers to such questions are not obvious. Perhaps that is part of what makes sports so glorious. The wisdom of the body's motor controllers that tick to an intrinsic clock. The athlete's experience and decision making. All of this coming together in a fascinating mélange that dictates athletic success.

These chapters present a recurring question: Is the control of physical effort over time—sport performance—under the conscious dictates of the athlete? That is, can runners in a 10K race willfully strategize their pace to produce the best result? Or, are they under the control of unconscious processes within their central nervous systems that decide, without their knowledge, how fast to go and how to regulate stride frequency and stride length? Do human beings control athletic performance or do forces of nature rule, such as rhythmic biological variations over time or inexorable deterioration with age over time?

If I could contact Charles Darwin on the bridge of the *Beagle*, I think I know how he would weigh in on this question. He'd say that the process of human locomotion has evolved over thousands of centuries, and the factors that define both the best way to move and the limits of physical exertion are the products of all that natural experimentation. These factors are geared toward survival—limits are placed to protect us from catastrophic outcomes (fatal dysrhythmias, bone fractures, shredded muscles), and we exercise in a way that best preserves energy stores.

And athletes? Even without a formal poll, we could predict that most would be skeptical of that argument. That athletes can't willfully strategize during a distance competition seems contrary to their experiences. Of course, this issue lies far beyond that simply of athletic success. It is quickly encountered by the end of the third week of any introductory philosophy course. Human determinism. Who (or what) is really in control here? The conscious or the subconscious? Are the forces of destiny—or the finish time in a 10K road race—under our conscious control?

Unlike the philosophical arguments, the question in the realm of athletic performance is at least potentially amenable to an experimental approach. The latter pages of this book examine some of these investigations. Even when nature is clearly a basic driving force—as in the effects of aging on performance—can athletes use cognitive strategies to subdue or overcome limits placed by biological factors that are out of their direct control? Is it safe to do so? I now count eight questions in the last three paragraphs without any obvious answers. Alas, insights to these dilemmas are not altogether at hand. But, such issues are intriguing. In many cases, they also have direct bearing on how athletes should best face competitive challenges.

But why write a book on this subject? In doing so, I have two particular goals in mind. The first is to examine some aspects of time that carry very real importance for performing athletes. How is muscular work best adjusted relative to time to provide optimal pacing during aerobic endurance competitions like distance running or cycling? How are such approaches changed when, instead of pacing, an all-out effort (such as in short-distance sprinting) is called for? Do particular times of day or season make sport training more effective or maximize performance? Can athletes alter their perception of time to improve neuromotor responses to high-speed events like, for instance, hitting a pitched baseball? Chapters 1, 3, 4, and 5 focus on these questions. Clearly, we are only beginning to understand these issues. But, it would seem that this information underscores the idea that understanding how time influences motor performance may offer valuable guidance to athletes. I hope this book will provide sport competitors with concrete strategies for optimizing athletic performance.

Do athletes perceive time differently than nonathletes? Consider the quarterback engineering an offensive drive in the final two minutes who is trailing by a touchdown. The returner of the serve at Wimbledon who is down a break in the fifth set. Do they feel time in a unique way? The answer is not entirely clear, but these pages may reveal some clues.

Beyond such issues, too, this book presents some fascinating questions regarding the basic mechanisms by which time influences physiological function, which then can be translated into pushing the limits of motor performance. The first three chapters examine how subconscious directors of motor activity within the central nervous system dictate how fast we run, and how the complex sequence of muscle activation and its tempo are best regulated for optimal performance. Chapter 4 addresses the intriguing biological clock that alters function in a temporal fashion. These circadian rhythms, first recognized for whole animals, are witnessed even at a molecular level in individual cells themselves. The final chapter reviews how, over the life span, time alters motor function, particularly as it decays in the waning years of life. It shows that the dictates of time are inexorably linked to the limits of human existence.

This book takes you on a journey through the effects of time on motor performance. It does so from the standpoint of how such an understanding might be utilized by athletes to improve performance. It also appreciates the incredible complexity and beauty—dare we call it spirituality?—that underlies such mechanisms. These, in effect, serve in many ways to define our existence on this planet. In doing so, then, John, I attempt to keep the magic.

Notes

1. A thorough discussion of the direction of time can be found in the following sources: Convency, R., and R. Highfred. 1990. *The arrow of time*. London: W.H. Allen. Leggett, A.J. 1982. "The 'arrow of time' and quantum mechanics." In *The enigma of time*, ed. P.T. Landsberg, 149-156. Bristol: Adam Hilger.

2. Philosophical (and sentimental) considerations of the nature of the passage of time can be found in this work: Pessoa, Fernando. 2002. *The book of disquiet*. London: Penguin Books.

3. There are a number of excellent and very readable reviews of the influence of body size on physiological function, including the following: Bonner, J.T. 2006. *Why size matters*. Princeton, NJ: Princeton University Press. Calder, W.A. 1984. *Size, function, and life history*. Cambridge, MA: Harvard University Press,

p. 141. Schmidt-Nielsen, K. 1984. *Scaling. Why is animal size so important?* Cambridge, MA: Cambridge University Press.

4. Further reading on biological maturation of physical fitness during growth: Malina, R.M., C. Bouchard, and O. Bar-Or. 2004. *Growth, maturation, and physical activity*. 2nd ed. Champaign, IL: Human Kinetics.

5. More on the randomness of streaks in athletic performance can be found in the following sources: Gilovich, T., R. Vallone, and A. Tversky. 1985. "The hot hand in basketball: On the misperception of random sequences." *Cognitive Psychology* 17: 295-314. Mlodinow, L. 2008. *The drunkard's walk. How randomness rules our lives*. New York: Vintage Books.

6. Price, V. 1994. "The other kingdom." In *The runner's literary companion*, ed. G. Battista, p. 66. New York: Penguin Books.

CHAPTER 1

Selecting the amount of muscle force to generate over time—race speed—is critical for optimizing performance in sports like distance running, cycling, and swimming. This chapter examines how such velocities are chosen, monitored, and adjusted—either by the athlete's cognition or by a clever mechanism located within the central nervous system that controls the subconscious.

WHO'S IN CHARGE HERE?

Setting the Race Pace

In the spring of 2008, on the Isle of Wight, a British photographer named Norman Potter put on an exhibition of 50 pieces of his work titled, rather mysteriously, "Photographer Unknown." Guests strolled about, taking in images of war, politicians, famine, and train robbers. Suddenly, on the back wall, there it was: without question, the greatest sports photo of all time. Roger Bannister, mouth agape and head thrown back, gasping for air in his final, agonizing strides to the tape in 3:59.4.

We see the spectators, some cheering, some frozen in awe. The timekeeper, maintaining his British cool, puffs on his pipe and soberly checks his stopwatch. The four-minute mile, incredibly, had been achieved! 5,280 feet. In fewer than 240 ticks of the clock. Some had said it would never happen. Others were worried that the human machine would fail before it went that fast. But here it was, the moment captured for eternity (figure 1.1).

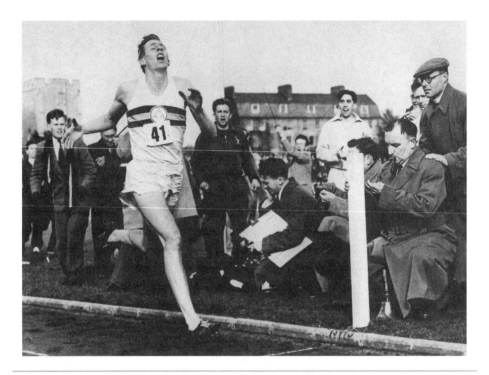

FIGURE 1.1. An iconic photo of Bannister breaking the four-minute-mile barrier.
PA Photos.

Norman Potter was the person who took that picture, but nobody knew it for 50 years. The greatest sports photo ever. It was always published with the credit line "photographer unknown" (thus explaining the exhibition title) or "central press." It wasn't until 2004 that Potter, by now a legendary photographer, revealed it to be his. He explained that in 1954, agency pictures were not usually attributed to individual photographers. And he was, after all, just a young press photographer at the time, starting out a five-year apprenticeship. "Photography did not make me rich or famous," he told a reporter from the *Isle of Wight News*, "but what a great life I've had." (In a parallel fashion, the original 5-by-4 inch glass negative of his famous photo had been missing for 20 years when it was discovered, with a large crack down the center, in a box of broken photo plates. Thanks to some technological tricks, it has now been restored.)

Potter's photo shows some other things, too: a return of dignity and self-respect to a war-torn Great Britain, a victory for what some considered the purity of amateur sport, a symbol of the power of the human will to overcome seemingly impossible barriers. It is a fitting start to the pages of this book, since there has been no greater monument to athletic sacrifices in response to the challenge of time.

Many are aware that Roger Bannister was a medical student at nearby Oxford during those heady days in the spring of 1954. Less well known, though, is that he was also completing a research scholarship on the physiology of running. Bannister was a researcher, and his insights into how the human machine responds to high-intensity exercise in the laboratory were crucial in formulating his plans for racing success.[1] He deduced that an important aspect was reducing energy demands, which could best be achieved by the following measures:

- Running as smoothly as possible
- Eliminating useless motion
- Keeping an even pace

He reasoned that during his mile attempt, he would lose more energy by accelerating than he would save by slowing down. Therefore, keeping his energy demands as constant as possible would be critical to his success. (His actual lap-split times in breaking the four-minute barrier were 57.5, 60.5, 62.4, and 59.0 seconds.)

Not a great deal has changed since then. The track on Iffley Road where the four-minute barrier was smashed is still used by Oxford students, though its dirt and cinder lanes are long gone. It has been renamed in Sir Roger's honor and paved over with an artificial surface. Sir Roger himself still lives in Oxford, just a few minutes away. He has completed a distinguished 40-year career as a neurologist, contributing important insights into why the autonomic nervous system sometimes fails to respond to stressful stimuli. Norman Potter is doing more fishing these days. The weather? Well, that's not changed much either—it's still gray, cool, windy, and drizzly. (It cleared, miraculously, just before Sir Roger's assault on the mile record.)

Half a century later, Potter's iconic photograph still sends a chill down the spine. It sets the stage for many of the ideas in this chapter—the scientific approach to pacing strategies, the question of who (or what) controls the limits of racing effort, and, not least, the importance of taking a good photo at the finish tape.

Optimal Pacing Strategy

When it comes to choosing strategies for performance success, football teams (the American variety, that is) have it made—they've a lot to choose from. Just before the snap of the ball, it's a mystery to the defense what it's going to be—a handoff up the middle, a screen pass, a running sweep around the end, a long pass on a post pattern, maybe even a quick kick. Basketball players might choose a fast break, a backdoor cut off a screen, a dunk from a low post (which could be countered by a shift to a zone defense), a trap, or a full-court press. Tennis players, too, have lots of options—a backhand down the line, a drop shot, a slice, a lob.

But, alas, not so for the runner, swimmer, or cyclist. In fact, there's not too much to choose from. The goal in these sports is to produce the greatest amount of muscular work per unit of time for a particular distance. In doing so, athletes have only the following choices:

- Producing a greater muscular effort over a shorter time (going faster)
- Reducing power output over a longer time (slowing down)
- Simply maintaining a constant velocity throughout (utter madness!)

Sure, during training, they can strategize by altering the timing, frequency, and distance of tempo runs; LSD (long, slow distance); and speed work. Dietary intake can be adjusted (carbohydrate loading), equipment can be manipulated, tapering schedules can be constructed, mental toughness can be developed, and legs can be shaven. But once the gun goes off, the only means of optimizing race success is to select (more about this later) the right rate of effort relative to time.

In optimizing, athletes need to run, swim, or cycle at a velocity that will deliver them to the finish line at just the critical point (before muscle-power production approaches a precipitous decline). The competitor in a 10K road race can't go out too fast. Researchers have actually studied this at its extremes. And, to no great surprise, studies in which subjects were told to go all out from the start on a treadmill or cycle, without a thought of slowing down, don't last long.

If you volunteer to perform a Wingate anaerobic cycling test, you'll be asked to give your all-out best effort for 30 seconds. What will happen? First, your top power output will last about 5 seconds, then fall off by about 50% by the end of the test at most. (Author's suggestion: Refuse to do this. You have at least a 70% chance of violent emesis at the finish.) These findings fit with what is seen in actual athletic competition. As we'll see in a later chapter, even in the brief moments of a 100-meter dash, the world's best sprinters can't maintain a maximal speed for more than 7 seconds. That's just a little more than half the duration of the event. So, here's the obvious moral: A maximal effort as the gun fires at the starting line of a distance race will be ruinous. For any event lasting more than 30 seconds or so, some kind of pacing—regulating a speed somewhere below a peak effort—is required.[2]

Here is another time experiment that you can try for yourself. At your next 10K road race, start at the front of the pack, right next to all those people who suspiciously resemble Steve Prefontaine.[3] When the gun goes off, sprint out just as fast as you can. Two things will happen. First, you will be engulfed by a wave of euphoria—you are actually leading the race! Two, the sensation will be quickly over. Inevitably, in a very short time, "Pre" and his buddies will all come rushing by you. The point of the experiment is to see how long that will take. (This author probably holds the minimum time record for western Massachusetts men over 60 of 7.63 seconds.)

On the other hand, an overly relaxed pace, in which athletes are not exhausted crossing the finish line, is equally daft. They shouldn't be able to walk back to the car with a set of fresh legs. Within these two extremes, distance athletes must take off at a particular speed that can be sustained, adjusting during the race as needed. This provides the greatest average-muscle work per time, leaving them truly exhausted at the finish line, but not before.

Exercise physiologists in testing laboratories have searched long and hard to discover just what determines a champion aerobic endurance athlete. But sport performance is a very complicated business. It remains an unsolved mystery which of the many metabolic, neuromuscular, cardiorespiratory, and psychological factors that go into muscular work capacity is responsible for limiting performance. But you would have to say that, such uncertainties notwithstanding, the answer is not of particular interest for athletes in the middle of a race. Instead, they must focus on finding a strategy of speed that provides the best performance within the setting of whatever anatomical or physiological limits exist at the time. So, training regimens can be constructed in response to research insights in an effort to improve their competitive success. When it comes to race day, though, their performance will rest on optimal pacing strategy.

Picking the Pace: Distance and Speed

So, which speed is best? How do athletes go about selecting the optimal velocity for starting a distance event? How can they then adjust their speed at different times during the event to ensure that their optimal degree of effort—the point of exhaustion—will coincide with crossing the finish line? These are key questions. Let's think about the answer from two different points of view. One is based on a traditional pacing model of cognitive responses to perception of effort. The athletes are in control—they consciously make pacing decisions. But there's another, rather intriguing explanation. It says that the central nervous system—your brain—subconsciously regulates muscle effort to give you your best performance. And it does this in the name of safety, protecting you from anatomical and physiological damage. It's sort of a wise and benevolent central governor.

Cognitive Pacing Strategy

Experienced distance athletes know how they feel during a race. From having competed in similar distances in the past, they know just how intense such perceptions of effort should be in order to predict exhaustion at the finish. Breathing too hard and experiencing leg-muscle stress in the first kilometer of a 10K race cause runners to conclude that they will not make it at this pace. They consciously slow their velocity. Conversely, being too comfortable in the early phases of a race signals them to speed up.

This traditional model of pacing is rooted in the idea that athletes make cognitive, purposeful decisions regarding running velocity based on previous experience and sensory input. But which cues do they use to make these velocity adjustments?

Exercise scientists measure how athletes feel as their *rating of perceived exertion* (RPE). Here, athletes report subjective sensations of exercise stress, usually on a numerical scale ranging from 6 to 20. (This is called a Borg scale, with the top number indicating the very highest level of fatigue.) This, then, is an attempt to put an objective measure (a number) to a subjective feeling ("How hard does it feel?"). Using this tool, the goal of researchers has been to identify the physiological (heart and lung function, body temperature), metabolic (blood acidity, lactate levels), and neuromuscular (muscle stress) factors that are most important in signaling the athletes' level of subjective stress during a distance competition. By monitoring all this input, then, competitors figure out how to adjust race velocity to provide their best effort for a particular competition distance.

However, which particular input cues are the most critical in this strategizing are not entirely clear. A whole variety is possible, but despite a good deal of research, physiologists remain pretty much in the dark as to exactly how the athlete senses level of effort. Heart rate, oxygen uptake, and rate and depth of breathing have all been linked to RPE, as have blood-lactate level, availability of blood sugar, body temperature, and blood or muscle pH (acidity). Since all of these factors are in fact altered with increased work intensity, however, it is difficult to determine which, if any, actually cause changes in RPE. (Author's note: An informal survey of running acquaintances would seem to confirm personal experience that the agonizing discomfort of labored breathing is the most prominent signal of stress in a 5K or 10K road race. Does it help to recognize that this gasping indicates that excessive carbon dioxide is building up in your blood during the buffering of lactic acid, which is now flooding out of your muscle cells? Nope. Not at all.)

You might think, too, that external cues, such as where you are in relation to other competitors, could be important. If you, the state cross country champion, are at the back of the pack, your pace is too slow. Split times, which are provided specifically to help competitors regulate velocity, should be expected to be particularly useful in regulating effort in a distance event. But, perhaps surprisingly, this conclusion has not always been supported by research findings.

For instance, Yumna Albertus and her colleagues at the University of Cape Town shamelessly deceived trained cyclists during 20K time trials to see if providing false split times would change their pacing strategy. On the first time trial, the split times were correct, but on the second trial, the first split was actually given at .775 kilometers. This was followed by an increase of 25 meters with each subsequent kilometer until the end, when the split was given at 1.25 kilometers. On a third trial, the fraudulent times were reversed. So, did all this trickery affect the cyclists' pacing strategy? Surprisingly, not at all. There were no differences in finish times among the three trials. RPE values were the same, too. In finding that the pattern of power output was similar during the three trials, the researchers could conclude that the pacing strategy didn't change, either. Their conclusion? Pacing strategy is regulated by intrinsic clues (how an athlete feels), rather than by distance feedback.[4]

Another investigation by Hugh Morton from New Zealand in which subjects were deceived produced different results. In this case, soccer players were asked to cycle to exhaustion (at a set resistance and cadence) on three occasions while facing a large digital clock. They didn't know that the clock was rigged to show the normal time on one occasion, to run 10% slower another time, and to run 10% faster the third. The results: When the clock ran slow, aerobic endurance time averaged 18% higher, compared to the session with normal time. There was no effect on aerobic endurance time, however, with the fast clock.

It was uncertain how to explain all this. The author himself was puzzled, concluding that "the psychological mechanisms behind the findings in this study are unclear."[4] But there does seem to be evidence here that external cues—in this case, the knowledge of time—are important in defining exercise tolerance. One conclusion is sure, though. If you are asked to be a subject in a pacing study, check the administrator's honesty first.

(The parallel to these deception studies in the real world of road racing obviously occurs when split times are erroneous because of inaccurately placed mile markers. This becomes evident when you find you've just passed the first-mile split, having shaved a full three minutes off the world record for this distance.)

This, then, is the customary way that coaches and distance athletes think about pacing. The competitors are in charge. They step up to the starting line, anticipating an average race speed based on previous events. Then, based on an awareness of how they feel, sensory input from the body's physiological state, plus extrinsic cues (split times), they modify their rate of muscular work (pace) during the race. These factors contribute to their optimal overall finishing time for that particular day and set of race conditions.

Subconscious Control by the Central Nervous System

An alternative view of pacing takes control of race pace out of the hands of the athlete and places it into the automatic, unconscious realm of the central nervous system. According to this model, the brain acts as a protector, or *governor*, regulating motor activity to keep the body safe. Here's how the story goes:

Viewed from a Darwinian perspective, your performance in a 5K road race, in addition to impressing your friends, is an evolutionary outcome that was originally linked to survival value—the capacity to acquire food and escape from enemies. In this context, it makes no evolutionary sense that intensive exercise should prove risky to the human organism.

But, in fact, there is no doubt that it certainly could be. With exhaustive levels of exercise, an athlete might overheat to the point of cardiorespiratory shock and death. Skeletal muscle could go into spasmodic contractions and shred. The same muscle has the ability to contract with sufficient force to break bones. As heart rate reaches high levels, the blood flow through the coronary arteries that supply the heart could be compromised. Intense contractions could trigger dangerous levels of heart muscle fatigue, predisposing the heart to abnormal, life-threatening rhythms. It's not a pretty picture.

The observation that such tragic events very rarely, if ever, occur was not lost on A.V. Hill and his colleagues, who suggested in 1924 that during high-intensity exercise, a governor "causes slowing of the circulation as soon as a serious degree of [oxygen] unsaturation occurs, since it would obviously be very dangerous for [the heart] to be able to exhaust itself very completely."[5] More recently, the idea that the brain communicates beneath the level of consciousness to prevent the risk of extreme exercise stress through signals of fatigue has been espoused and developed by others, particularly Tim Noakes and his colleagues in South Africa.[5] They believe that "there is no evidence that homeostatic control fails at exhaustion in any form of exercise. . . . In contrast, the single variable that is always maximal at exhaustion during all forms of exercise is the rating of perceived exertion."

The idea here is that those miserable feelings of fatigue that cause an athlete to slow down or stop are just that: feelings, perceptions, sensations, rather than specific physiological or metabolic markers. They come from the central nervous system, and they are the brain's way of preventing you from exercising beyond the limits of safety. According to this explanation, then, the velocity sustained during a distance race is not dictated by an athlete's cognitive selection, but rather by the brain. It establishes the fastest pace, the greatest amount of muscular work over time that is safe for that particular distance.

By this concept, this subconscious, protective brake limits exercise by two means. First, it reduces *central command*, the signals descending down the spinal cord from the brain to the contracting muscle that control strength of contractions. And, second, it creates that familiar set of agonizing feelings we call *fatigue*, which for most of us makes further effort intolerable. In this way, such feelings are a symptom created by a guardian central nervous system, rather than a physiological or physical state.

This is not to say that physiological or metabolic factors are not critical determinants of performance. They are, and it is from these variables that the brain gets its input to decide which rate of muscular work is safe. According to the central governor hypothesis, though, it's those conscious sensations of fatigue themselves—projected from a subconscious controller—that limit aerobic endurance performance.

If you think about it, what ultimately limits your abilities in a 10K road race? Is it not those unpleasant feelings of fatigue that eventually become quite intolerable? Ask subjects who have just completed a treadmill test to exhaustion why they had to stop. They'll probably have trouble putting it into words, but the idea will be that they just felt "devastated." (British participants will feel "shattered," French will be "crevées.")

The operant word here is *felt*. This set of sensations obviously arose in the conscious brain. When the subjects reached a maximal effort on the treadmill, their hearts were not damaged from lack of blood flow, their leg muscles weren't in spasm, their brains were not fried, their bones were not broken. In fact, their lungs were functioning at about 70% of peak capacity. Instead, they stopped because they felt bad.

The critical question here is did those sensations arise, as traditionally assumed, from the physiological and metabolic consequences of high-intensity exercise (lactic acid accumulating in the bloodstream, elevated body temperature, depletion of energy fuels like glycogen)? Or, do the exercise-limiting sensations of fatigue arise from the unconscious portions of the brain which, having sensed physiological information indicating high-exercise stress, depress force of muscle contraction and block the desire to continue, all in the name of preserving safety (figure 1.2)?

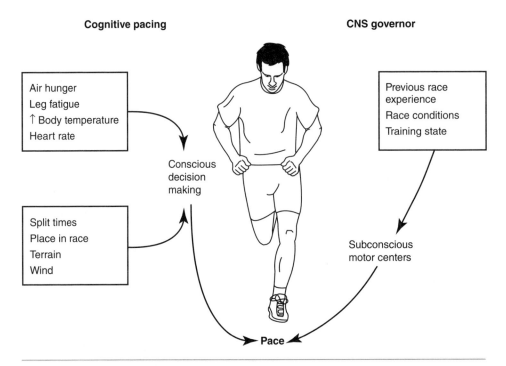

FIGURE 1.2. What controls race velocity in distance running? Do you have a say (the cognitive approach, listening to sensory signals)? Or does an unconscious brain governor dictate pace to optimize performance while looking out for your safety?

Which one is correct? How can we tell the difference? One way would be to examine situations in which feelings of fatigue and the inability to continue to exercise become dissociated, or separated, from maximal physiological or metabolic measures. That is, if we could demonstrate that sensations of a peak effort do not always coincide with certain factors, such as maximal utilization of oxygen by the muscles, peak heart rate, blood lactic acid levels, and elevations in core temperature, we would have evidence supporting the idea that fatigue during a distance event is primarily a subconscious brain process, rather than a physiological event. In fact, a number of pieces of such evidence do exist:

● One way to demonstrate that feelings of fatigue can be dissociated from physiological markers is by administering certain drugs. For example, it has been demonstrated that subjects given naloxone, which blocks actions of mood-elevating endorphins in the brain, stop exercising earlier because of high RPE (rating of perceived exertion) values, even though their oxygen uptake, heart rate, and ventilation were far from maximal values. This suggests that exercise capacity is determined by perception of effort rather than by physiological limitations.

● When a person exercises at high altitude or in conditions of low ambient oxygen, the capacity for aerobic endurance is reduced. However, at the point of exhaustion, athletes may not always reach their limits of heart and lung function or metabolic capacity. For example, cardiac output during peak exercise with 15% inspired oxygen (compared to the usual 20%) is approximately 10% lower than in normal conditions. Noakes' group asserts that this observation supports the existence of a brain governor that protects the heart (and brain, too) from hypoxia and ischemic damage.

● Researchers have manipulated respiratory effort by having subjects breathe against resistance during exercise, fooling the brain into thinking that exercise effort was increasing. The result: Exercise tolerance was decreased. Subjects stopped due to fatigue, with a heart rate well beneath the expected maximal value and with no evidence of weakness in leg muscles.

● Exercise is commonly depressed in the heat, compared to cool, ambient temperatures. Dehydration and limitations in blood circulation may contribute to this effect, but when subjects remain normally hydrated, diminished aerobic endurance in the heat is not accompanied by evidence of cardiorespiratory compromise. Instead, it appears that exercise performance in the heat is limited by inhibitory effects of fatigue from the central nervous system in response to a rise in core (or brain) temperature. This brain brake may thereby prevent excessive exercise that poses risks of heatstroke, cardiorespiratory collapse, renal failure, and breakdown of muscle tissue (rhabdomyolysis).

This collective body of evidence provides at least some indirect support for the concept that a brain governor limits the intensity or duration of exercise "to ensure homeostasis is maintained and catastrophe averted." And, on reflection, this is really not a novel idea. Indeed, it seems almost trite to point out the myriad of similar protective, controlling mechanisms that exist to maintain the constancy of the body systems (the great 19th-century physiologist Claude Bernard termed this the "milieu intérieur"). Appetite and thirst centers protect us from dehydration and low blood sugar. Thermoregulatory mechanisms maintain the cell in a delicately narrow temperature range. The kidney tubules, through selective secretion and absorption, maintain a constant composition of blood electrolytes, and so on. These many feedback controllers, which are critical to existence, are all performed below the level of consciousness. It should come as no surprise that we are protected against hyperthermia, myocardial damage, and muscle rigor as intense exercise is performed over time.

But, the discerning reader will protest, how would such a subconscious brain velocity controller set an appropriate pace at the start of a distance race, before any sensory input is available? This is where the concept of the central governor takes a fascinating turn. It has been proposed that, based on a bank of knowledge of past experience, the central controller recognizes which rate of muscular effort can be safely expended for a particular distance or time. In response, this velocity is set at the beginning of the race. That is, the anticipatory governor acts toward a preprogrammed endpoint based on previous experience.

So, here I am at the starting line of the 10K road race. My brain is saying, "Okay, based on past experience, I calculate that my guy here can run this distance without throwing up, suffering a fatal episode of heart arrhythmia, developing a dangerous rise in core temperature, or generally disgracing himself if he goes at a pace of x minutes per mile. I will set his leg motor oscillator (see chapter 2) at a stride frequency and length to achieve this velocity at the start of the race. This should safely deliver him across the finish line in his best time."

"Ah," I hear you saying. "A hidden controller in the central nervous system with anticipatory powers that I'm not even aware of. Sorry, but that's a bit fantastic. Maybe even surreal." But, in fact, this idea is entirely in keeping with contemporary concepts of brain function that have been developed by our neurophysiological colleagues. Specifically, current trends in the field of cognitive neuroscience view brain activity as processing in a more proactive, top-down manner, rather than simply reacting to sensory input in a reflex fashion (from the bottom up).

The German neurobiologist Andreas Engel has written about the need to abandon simplistic, classical views of the brain "as a passive, stimulus-driven device that does not actively create meaning by itself."[6] (That's the model of the cognitive approach to pacing. The incoming signal to the brain at the 2-mile mark is that you're breathing too fast, prompting you to send signals to the muscles to slow the pace.) Instead, he describes a "paradigm shift" that considers the brain as able to predict future events and to act based on prior information. It controls actions even in advance of sensory input, a function that has been repeatedly observed in human and animal studies.

Engels states that this ability to predict and act independently of direct environmental cues, based on previous experience, "has been acquired both during evolution and through experience-dependent learning, and has proven to be of adaptive value." Thus, Engel would agree that there is a Darwinian advantage for the brain to be an in-charge decision maker that is not simply a slave to reflex responses in reaction to sensory input from the environment.[6] Sound familiar? Yes, this whole idea, which has been derived far removed from the arena of competitive athletics, is not altogether different from the idea of a protective, central governor that regulates aerobic endurance pacing. And all for the purpose of maintaining the integrity of body structure and function.

Where's the Proof?

If the subconscious brain controls pace, it must have the ability to closely monitor the passage of time. Such a central controller cannot operate effectively unless it is aware of the distance you've run and the time that's passed in the race. That means we must have, in all of us, a reliable, internal clock. This, then, is our first encounter in these pages of intrinsic timekeeping mechanisms, clocks that dictate exercise performance. Before we reach the end, we will find evidence for many more.

The central governor hypothesis, at least to my way of thinking, has a nice ring to it. I particularly like the way its homeostatic, protective function makes sense from the standpoint of biological evolution. It fits with contemporary notions of the controlling, rather than the passive, nature of brain function. To my mind, the process of evolution, of natural selection, would not allow a brain to be developed that would permit us to push ourselves into a realm of high risk. Trying to prove its ability to anticipate and control race pace, however, is another matter. Not an easy task.

I have yet to encounter a distance athlete who does not voice disbelief, if not outright disdain, for the idea that an unconscious brain governor controls pace during a race. That they are not in charge does not seem consistent with their experience. The same might be said of sports scientists, who have been generally slow to embrace this idea. Instead, they have voiced a good deal of skepticism. In 2009, Roy Shephard wrote a commentary titled "Is It Time to Retire the 'Central Governor'?" in which he claimed there was a "lack of convincing evidence" supporting the concept.[5] This opinion was shared by the majority of exercise scientists involved in a literary debate on the subject in the pages of the *Journal of Applied Physiology*. Reading through their input, I was impressed that it wasn't that they thought the idea was wrong, it was just that only insufficient evidence could be mustered, in their minds, to support it. And, in some cases, reasonable counter arguments were made supporting the traditional model of physiological and metabolic determinants of exercise performance. As Shephard concluded in his article, which pretty much summarized the debate itself, "until there is convincing experimental evidence of an underlying physiological mechanism, most sports scientists will continue to express skepticism concerning the existence of a 'central governor.'"

If this were 1890, one person, without doubt, would have stood up and vehemently supported the central governor hypothesis. Indeed, it was Sigmund Freud himself who opened the world's vision to the hubbub of deterministic mental activity that churned in our brains beneath the conscious level. His ideas, of course, generated a whole new way of looking at conscious behavior as an expression of repressed, subconscious processes. Alas, Freud's version of the central governor was not quite so benevolent as the one during exercise (proposed by Professors Hill and Noakes), instead taking repressed, subconscious feelings of unacceptable guilt, sexual fantasy, and psychological conflict and turning them into clinical mental disease.

Implications for the Athlete

In the meantime, what does all this business about a central governor mean to the distance athlete, who basically considers the sensations of fatigue as a barrier to optimal performance? Putting up with the

Riddle of Zeno's Paradox

You might wonder if the philosopher Zeno had any idea what a conundrum he was creating when he presented his *Paradox* in the year 450 BC. It puzzled great thinkers, setting the stage for many centuries of uncertain discussions and proposed solutions. Indeed, it's not clear even today that philosophers and mathematicians have a firm grasp on its explanation. Here's how it goes:

The warrior Achilles was challenged to a 1,500-meter race by Tortoise, who is, of course, a turtle. Achilles, recognizing his great speed advantage and being a good sport, tells the turtle that he will grant him a 100-meter head start. "In that case," says the turtle, "we don't have to run the race. There is no way that you can win." Stupefied, Achilles listens to the turtle's explanation.

"When the gun goes off, we'll both start running. You will quite quickly reach the 100-meter mark, where I started. But by that time, I will have gone farther than that, maybe to the 110-meter point. In the next moments, you will arrive there, but by then I will have run ahead to the 114-meter point. And this will continue. Every time you catch up to the spot where I was, I will have advanced in the race. Therefore, it is impossible for you to pass me. You cannot, in fact, win the race. You will always be behind. All I have to do to win the race is to keep running."

We recognize, of course, that this is false, since our common experience is that Achilles will win easily. Indeed, with a little mathematics, based on the velocities of the two competitors, it can be accurately calculated as to when and by how much Achilles will be the victor. Of course. But what is wrong with the turtle's reasoning? That's not quite so easy to say. You get the feeling something is fishy here, because in the turtle's scenario, the race would actually never end. His description requires progressively smaller units of time-distance measure, which would reach infinity, never achieving the finish. But we know that the race will, in fact, end.

We are left here with a paradox of two possibilities, both of which seem genuine. But if one is true, it would make the other impossible. The answer, unfortunately, is not in the back of this book. However, if you want to read more about Zeno and his paradox, here are some fascinating books:

Baggani, J. 2005. *The Pig That Wants to Be Eaten*. New York: Plume.
Mazur, J. *Zeno's Paradox*. 2007. New York: Plume.

pain, in effect, is viewed as a key to success in high-level sports. (As the German cyclist Gerald Ciolek commented when asked in a television interview how to survive the Tour de France, "Just shut off your head and go.") The research data suggests this is, in fact, true, that maximal exercise is limited by perceptual barriers and that all peak human performance is submaximal. But it also suggests that the athlete encroaches on such levels of exercise over the dictates of a knowledgeable central nervous system that is geared toward preventing intense, sustained muscular efforts that might pose a risk.

It is tempting to suggest that, with at least one exception, the margin of safety is sufficiently wide that even the most dedicated athlete can endeavor to push the limits of fatigue and discomfort. As witnessed by the anguished finishers in Olympic distance events, even the most exaggerated levels of muscular effort by otherwise healthy individuals don't result in myocardial infarction, fatal dysrhythmias, uncontrolled seizures, shattered bones, or shredded muscles. The exception seems to be the real risk associated with exhaustive performance in conditions when body temperature rises to dangerous levels. It's rare, but for some people, the central governor gets lulled or overcome. Well-documented examples exist of athletes who have suffered heat stroke with cardiorespiratory shock, or even death. Use of ergogenic aids may exacerbate such risks. An example is the tragic death of cyclist Tom Simpson from hyperthermia. He was climbing Mt. Ventoux on a hot day during the 1967 Tour de France. Sadly, postmortem findings and a later search of his hotel room revealed that he had consumed amphetamines during the race.

Professor Noakes has this to say on the subject: "The evidence has to be that the brain will prevent damage 99.999999999% of the time. When it 'fails,' it seems to me it is because there is pathology present—such as abnormal thermogenesis in muscle—which we may not understand. Having run so many marathons and been present so often at those races and at Iron triathlons, I simply don't see much evidence for 'failure'."

But can the central governor get things wrong? Can athletes underperform as a result? "The point of the central governor is to ensure that there is always a reserve," he says. "So, in a sense, it always promotes underperformance. Even in the world's best performances, there is still a reserve—the athletes could have gone faster. That is why they don't die at the finish."

Numbers back up these statements. Believers in human sanity will be shocked, but each year in the United States, almost half a million people participate in marathon races. Each one is trying to defy the limits of their central brain governor. What happens to all those people? In the end, not much. Sure, thousands visit the first-aid tent afterwards, but the consequences are typically minor and transient. It is estimated that American marathons lead to only four to six deaths each year. These are due to preexisting conditions (coronary artery disease, heart muscle abnormalities, congenital defects of the coronary arteries) or low blood sodium that results from drinking too much water.

This is true even in those remarkably rare cases of elite athletes who die during competition. Ryan Shay, for instance, tragically collapsed and died at the 5-mile (8 km) mark of the 2007 U.S. Olympic marathon trials. Autopsy revealed thickening and scarring of his heart muscle.

But what about heatstroke, the life-threatening rise in body temperature? Deaths from hyperthermia have occurred in distance races. Nonfatal cases are, of course, much more common. These are typically seen in shorter, high-intensity races. Each August, the medical tent at the 11.5-kilometer Falmouth Road Race on Cape Cod treats one or two cases for every 1,000 entrants. Bill Roberts, who has been medical director of the Twin Cities Marathon for the past 25 years, comments:

> According to the central control model, a central governor of activity should prevent an exercising person from developing exertional heatstroke by causing the athlete with hyperthermia affecting the brain to "fall out" of activity. Highly motivated athletes may be able to override the protective function of the central governor, and that can allow high levels of core organ overheating and eventual collapse.

Heatstroke might be expected in races conducted in hot, humid conditions in which highly motivated competitors are at risk for dehydration, but this is not always the case. For example, during the 2001 Chicago Marathon, a runner died with a core body temperature of 107 degrees F (42 degrees C), despite drinking fluids regularly during the race. The ambient temperature was only 50 degrees F (10 degrees C). Such observations have led some to believe, like Professor Noakes, that those occurrences of heatstroke in which the brain's controlling center is overridden by the athlete represent the effects of certain predisposing conditions, such as lack of heat acclimatization, viral illness, use of medication, or hereditary conditions leading to hyperthermia.[7]

Picking the Pace:
Selecting the Pattern of Speed

So far in this chapter, we've discussed how to best come up with an average speed (the work achieved per unit of time) required to get from point A to point B, a fixed distance. But we've been ignoring another aspect that's equally critical—how the velocity is parceled out during the journey. Indeed, some type of pacing strategy (how to vary or maintain speed during the race) is important for any event lasting more than 30 seconds. In this section, then, we'll examine how pacing strategy—selecting the pattern of speed—can affect performance.

Now we're getting to the part that makes distance racing really interesting, at least for the spectator. Pacing strategy, last-minute kicks, surges and challenges, duels and record-setting times. Without this, racing on the track would consist entirely, as they say in auto racing, of "a series of left turns." And out on the road, it would only interest those with TDFS (Tour de France syndrome), a peculiar affliction suffered by millions each July, in which otherwise innocent people are willing to sit on the side of a French road for three days to watch their favorite cyclist zip by in three to five seconds.

In the real world of competitive distance sports, of course, extrinsic factors play a dominant role in deciding pacing strategies: the distance of the race, weather conditions (temperature, wind), terrain (hills), personal strengths (a good finishing kick), knowledge of the opponents, and so on. But this section discusses—all things being equal—which tactics in varying pace during a distance race make the best sense. Call them models of prudent pacing, if you will. We'll look at common practices, explore a little bit of the limited data scientists have to offer on the subject, and, finally, learn the pacing strategies of successful athletes.

You can envision all sorts of patterns of velocity change during a distance race. But for this discussion at present, let's limit ourselves mainly to just three, which are diagrammed in figure 1.3. You can start fast, then try to hang on as velocity slows late in the race (line A). Or you can select an overall average pace you (or perhaps your uncon-

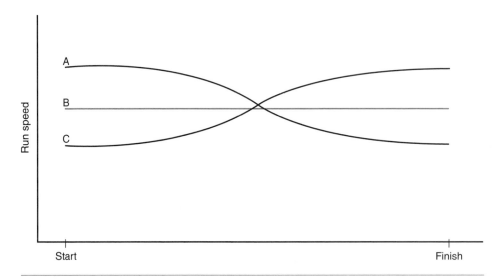

FIGURE 1.3. Three possible race-pacing strategies: As in A, start fast but finish slow; as in B, maintain a steady pace throughout; or as in C, race with a relaxed start and strong finish.

scious brain) desire to finish in, start out that way, and keep it steady throughout (line B). And (line C), you can start slow, but give it a big surge in the last mile or two, and maybe a kick at the end.

As you look at this figure, it is not altogether obvious that any one of these pacing strategies should be better than the others. Within reasonable variability, you might expect that the total work per distance is the same for all three options. Thus, to the uninitiated, it would seem that finish times would be equally similar. But that's not the way coaches and athletes have looked at it. In fact, selecting a particular pacing strategy has been considered a prime strategy for optimal success. But which one should you choose?

Many have advocated that best overall time can be accomplished in distance events with even pacing—keeping a steady split time (line B). They reason that steady pacing uses energy more economically, minimizes accumulation of lactic acid, prevents early drain of glycogen reserves (in long races), and delays detrimental rises in body temperature. Others have felt that aerobic endurance athletes are better off if they *negatively split*—completing the second half of the race slightly faster than the first. There might be some psychological value to this slow-fast approach (line C) in that the athlete would presumably feel better at a point that is closer to the end of the race.

Some say that a slightly faster start (line A) is better. But most would agree that jumping out with an overly fast start is a common error for distance athletes. It's hard to refrain from doing this—the gun goes off, adrenaline levels are sky high, the pack is moving fast, and you think that some early fast splits will put time in the bank, building a cushion for the inevitable slowdown when fatigue hits later on. On this, the experts are in accord—it doesn't work.

When you actually examine how elite runners perform, though, you commonly see a fairly rapid pace in the first portion of the race, a decline in the middle, and then a spurt at the end. This U-shaped pattern is particularly common in distances like the 1,500 meters, in which runners typically slow during the second and third laps but accelerate near the finish.

The best overall advice, then, seems to be to not stray very far from a constant velocity. How close should the chosen speed be? Some have used a 2% rule to guide pacing strategies for distance running. It states that the speed of a single split, including the first leg, should not deviate more than 2% (either faster or slower) from the desired overall pace for the race finish. Let's say you want to finish a 10K road race in 44:00, which means an average split time of 7:05 per mile

(1.6 km). According to this rule of thumb, your split time at the first mile should not deviate from this pace by more than 9 seconds. If your first-mile split is 6:54, slow down. If it's 7:18, speed up (but don't make up the entire difference in the very next mile). It is best to do these calculations before the race. It is common to find it difficult to perform math during actual competition. More likely than not, you'll forget something important, like carrying the one.

What do really good runners think about all this? To find out, I talked with a couple of them. One is newly on the scene, the other an experienced veteran. What they told me shows that racing strategies might be a bit different at the elite level. And, interestingly, their comments—despite their age difference of decades—were remarkably similar.

Paul Norton is an engaging young man who started running when he was in the seventh grade and has now blossomed into one of the top collegiate distance runners in the New England area. When we met for breakfast on a rainy morning at the Esselon Café on Route 9, he had just finished in seventh place in the Division III national cross country meet.

> At the start of a cross country race, I try to sprint out quickly—you don't want to get stuck up behind the other 250 runners. But after that, it's rapidly getting into a regular pace. In an 8K cross country race, it's not really time that's important, but rather finish place. You know those other guys and what they can do: who will challenge you, who won't. So, for the first two-thirds of the race, I'm just keeping it steady: sizing up the rest of the pack, keeping within striking distance. At this point, you really shouldn't be racing. I just try to stay comfortable—sort of zoned out. I watch a lot of runners put in surges early on, but that's just a lot of wasted energy.
>
> Then with a mile or two to go, the race really begins. I'm not sure I know just how I speed up. I just begin to gain momentum mentally. I think my brain is just subconsciously saying, "I'm going to catch those guys!"

Paul introduced me to an idea I hadn't thought of before—mental pacing. "Just like you have to regulate your physical effort to not become exhausted too early in a race, you have to conserve your mental effort. You only have so many physical and mental reserves. The end of the race will be tough. You have to have enough mental toughness left to push hard. That means staying really relaxed early on."

Mozart has a lot to do with Paul's success, too. In fact, Wolfgang A. was not particularly distinguished by his 10K times, but he sure knew how to keep a steady beat. Paul knows all about that. You see, he's a cellist, majoring in music performance at Brandeis (along with economics), and he loves chamber music. "For me, the big thing in racing is keeping a rhythm, keeping a constant effort. So, even pacing doesn't mean keeping the same times for all the splits, but rather maintaining the same effort. My legs are moving like a metronome, and what happens to me is that I get them moving in rhythm with some music in my head. It could be anything. Maybe the Mozart *Clarinet Quintet*, or even some Miley Cyrus the girls were singing on the bus. It helps me keep a constant stride cadence and pattern to my breathing."

During a race, I asked, does time flow any differently in your mind? "For sure! The 24:43 during an 8K cross country race (his personal best) is a lot longer than the 25 minutes spent eating this French toast. When I get tired, time just stretches out. That last mile—whew! 'Where is that finish line? When is this thing going to end?'" (Author's note: This verbal mantra is about the only running experience that Paul and I share.).

Jack Mahurin's days of burning up the track at Western Kentucky are well past, but he can look back with pride on a distinguished distance-running career. The highlight was a 12th place finish in the Boston Marathon in 1973, accomplished in 2:25 on blistering day of 80 degrees F (27 degrees C). "At the 10-mile (16 km) mark, I must have been in 800th place, but then people just started dropping like flies. I was conserving my energy stores, and I just started running by people." Impressive, too, is the fact that for four consecutive years at the height of his running, he put in an average of 100 training miles (160 km) a week without serious injury. Jack is now a physician, directing a family medicine program in Montgomery, Alabama. He still runs 30 miles (48 km) a week, but no longer races. His resting heart rate is 32 beats per minute.

> Much of my decision about how fast to run the first part of a race was simply an extension of what I did in training. The training was critical. That is, I learned what my speed should be in my daily sessions during the week, and then on race day, I simply went out and did it.
>
> The real challenge came near the end of the race. You don't want to be worrying about your times or winning or anything like that before then. There's only one statistic that counts—your finish time. So I would just try to keep in touch with the other guys early on, sort of sit on their shoulder, then try to hammer them as we approached the finish.
>
> The key for me was not to lose my technique. Just keep a relaxed rhythm. And I would think about those things a lot during the race. How I was feeling, how my legs were moving, what hills were coming up, the

weather, the next water stop. No time for daydreaming. I just concentrated a lot.

Pacing in Other Sports

Cycling has another school of thought on this matter. In a middle-distance event, you ought to blast off at the start with an all-out effort to bring yourself to the desired, submaximal race pace as quickly as possible. The argument goes like this: Yes, a steady cycling pace is best, and any deviation is energy expensive. So, the sooner that steady pace is reached, the better. An all-out initial start with rapid acceleration minimizes the time of transition to that desired pace. That is, the steady pace can thus be maintained for a longer period of time. There is also evidence that an all-out start is advantageous in rapidly gearing up the aerobic metabolic machinery.

Mathematical models and some experimental data also support this idea. The efficacy of this approach has mainly been demonstrated in cycling time trials between 30 seconds and 5 minutes, in which competitors put forth a top effort for the first 5% of the event. As noted by Brad Aisbett and his fellow researchers at Queensland University of Technology, however, "a near maximal starting effort must quickly give way to a more sustainable pace or fatigue will rapidly ensue."[8]

In swimming competitions in distances greater than 100 meters, there is even more reason to suggest that a steady pace is best. The work of a swimmer consists largely of overcoming the resistance created as the body moves through the water. Water resistance varies by the square of the swimmer's velocity. When swimmers increase their speed from 2 feet (60 cm) per second to 4 feet (122 cm) per second, the resistance doesn't double. Rather, it rises fourfold. The message: Speeding up costs the swimmer a good deal of extra energy.

So, in distance-swimming competitions, the general recommendation has been to keep as even a pace as possible throughout the race, saving whatever energy might remain for a sprint at the end. Some elite swimmers, however, have adopted a strategy of negative splitting (Janet Evans did this), swimming the first part of races at a slightly slower speed. Below the top level of competitors, however, most swimmers take off at a pace that is too fast, leading to progressive slowing and deterioration from fatigue in the later phases of the race.

Rowers, well, they've got a pacing plan all their own. In a typical 2,000-meter event, which lasts 6 to 8 minutes, the boat sets out at a vigorous pace at the starting signal. The stroke rate is something like 50 per minute, and it lasts about 30 to 45 seconds. This all-out burst is designed to overcome inertia and get the boat up to speed. Then, in the middle of the race, the velocity slows somewhat to a steady state of 35 to 40 strokes per minute. This continues until about a minute before the end, when a sprint to the finish occurs, an all-out effort that uses whatever energy remains.

An analysis of events in the Olympic Games and World Championship competitions showed that on the average, boats covered the first 500 meters 5.1 seconds faster than the second 500, with a small surge at the finish. This jump start is even more remarkable when you remember that the boats take off from a stationary position. It has been suggested that the power required by the rowers to accelerate the boat from zero to race pace may be as much as twice that required to cover the same distance at steady pace later in the race. Why do they do this? Besides overcoming boat inertia, getting out to a quick lead may offer advantages from a tactical standpoint, since the rowers can see the other boats and can also avoid their wake.[9]

Physiologically, this opening sprinting strategy doesn't make much sense. As the boat dashes away from the start, there's not enough time for muscles to gear up their aerobic (oxygen-using) metabolism, so the muscle cells have to resort to obtaining energy from anaerobic metabolism, building up a lot of lactic acid. And that makes muscles tired. Maybe that's why this sport is so physically demanding. (Crew is also set apart as being one of only three competitive sports events in which the winner finishes facing backwards. Here's a trivia question: What are the other two? The answer is in the notes at the end of the chapter.[10])

As an aside, it is perhaps worth noting that athletes might be skeptical of conforming to experts' recommendations of how it should be done. Indeed, some of the world's most talented athletes have performed with major departures from expected techniques. Bob Feller kicked up to heaven before delivering his fast ball, and Luis Tiant looked at second base. Dick Fosbury high-jumped over the bar backward (gasp!), and Bill Koch skated on cross-country skis.

Perhaps the best example, though, was the ungainly gait of the great Czech runner Emil Zàtopek (figure 1.4). Considered one of the greatest distance runners of the 20th century, Zàtopek accomplished the unheard-of feat of winning gold medals in all three of the distance-running events at the 1958 Olympic Games in Helsinki: the 5,000-meter, 10,000-meter, and marathon races. But today's coaches would hesitate to show their young runners films of Zàtopek running. This was the way not to do it! His upper and lower body went in opposite directions, swaying from side to side, while his head rolled and his face contorted in an agonizing effort (figure 1.4). He wheezed so loudly he was given the nickname "the Czech locomotive." Larry Snyder, track coach at Ohio State, reportedly said that "he does everything wrong but win."

What Research Tells Us

Is there any science behind all this advice about pacing strategy? Considering the supposed importance of proper pacing to performance, surprisingly little. For those wishing the details, here's a quick overview of what the research data tell us:

Much reference has been made to an early study by Sid Robinson that described findings of two middle-distance runners during three separate three-minute treadmill runs of even, fast-slow, and slow-fast paces. Performance was actually not addressed in this study. Instead, it focused on the body's rate of oxygen consumption, or efficiency, during each segment of the run. The assumption was that a greater efficiency (lower oxygen uptake per minute) might translate into better performance. Both subjects showed the worst efficiency with the fast-slow pattern. One showed optimal efficiency with a steady pace and the other with slow-fast.

In another part of that study, the authors demonstrated dramatic rises in both oxygen demand and blood lactate concentration in the terminal phases of a three-minute run. The authors stated, then, that to save on energy demands during a race, athletes should avoid early fatigue and refrain from running faster than the average, desired overall pace. The former

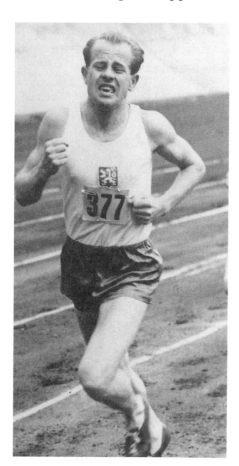

FIGURE 1.4. No one would suggest imitating Emil Zàtopek's running style.

AP Photo

would be achieved by starting off a little slower than the average speed to delay fatigue and permit a fast finish. The latter was best satisfied by maintaining an even pace throughout. In any case, a rapid start was not a good idea.

However, a similar study in 10 middle- and long-distance runners came to the opposite conclusion. Subjects ran with a fast-slow, slow-fast, or steady pace for 1,400 meters in four minutes on a treadmill. The fast-slow protocol resulted in lower lactate levels, faster rise in $\dot{V}O_2$ (that's good), and lower RPE during the final two minutes. No differences in muscle efficiency were observed among the three runs.

And then there is the study that examined the effects of a fast start on 5K running times in female distance runners. For the first 1.63 kilometers, subjects ran paces that were even, 3% faster, and 6% faster than a previously determined average race pace. By statistical analysis, the overall 5K racing times for the three patterns were not different, but a trend was observed for better times with the start that was 6% faster (averages were 2:11, 20:52, and 20:39 for the even start, the one that was 3% faster, and the one that was 6% faster, respectively). It was concluded that a fast-slow strategy was not detrimental to performance for 5K race times, and that a start with a speed increase of 3 to 6% might be advised.

Hettinga and colleagues had nine cyclists perform three 1,500-meter ergometer time trials with even, fast-slow, and slow-fast strategies. No differences in oxygen (energy) demand were observed in the three patterns. The research team headed by Carl Foster found that among five pacing strategies, an even pace resulted in the fastest overall time for a 2K cycling time trial performed in the laboratory. However, when they extended their observations to speed skaters in 1,500-meter competitions, this conclusion wasn't supported. Instead, the findings suggested that faster overall times were associated with a more rapid start.

In swimming, Thompson and colleagues showed that an even pace in 175-meter breaststroke time trials resulted in lower blood lactate levels after exercise, lower RPE, and greater variability of turn times compared to positive or negative pacing. These findings notwithstanding, they noted that positive pacing was employed by most national and international 200-meter breaststroke swimmers.

In cycling, competitors seem to have a tendency to initiate time trials with a greater power output than the desired average for the event. Some evidence shows that they can improve performance times by avoiding this energetic start. By mathematical models, it has been suggested, too, that cyclists are best off increasing power when pedaling uphill or against the wind, then reducing power in downhill sections or when traveling with a tailwind.

In simulated road races with treadmill running in the laboratory, however, the increased metabolic cost of running uphill has been found to be greater than the reduction when descending the same hill. This would imply that it would be wise to refrain from pushing too hard on the upslope, and then try to speed up on the descent.[11]

It would seem obvious from this small smattering of diverse studies that science is currently not a big help in defining optimal pacing strategies for distance athletes. Results are often conflicting, and it is questionable just how many of such laboratory findings can be translated to the real world of distance racing. In fact, small, statistically insignificant differences among a limited number of research subjects might be critical to performance in distance events in which a few seconds could bear real importance.

Picking the Pace: Doing as They Do

It would seem, then, that athletes and their coaches have always been a bit skeptical about embracing scientific data on pacing strategies, which, they might suggest, are a bit removed from the real world of racing. Instead, they've banked on their own experiences. We might well examine, then, some pacing lessons we could learn from distance runners.

Pull a Surprise

In the mid-1800s, distance running was performed by professionals, particularly in England. Called *pedestrians*, they would run all sorts of distances, with hefty wagers riding on the results. The pacing strategy was pretty much the same for every event. The runners would clump together at a comfortable, moderate pace for the duration of the race and then would make a mad sprint just as they approached the finish line (not unlike today's distance cyclists).

Enter upon this scene a native American named Deerfoot (actually Lewis Bennett) from western New York. He arrived in England in the fall of 1861 to challenge the Brits in a series of races of 4 to 10 miles (6-16 km). Going for a psychological advantage even before the start, he would appear at the track in full Seneca regalia—headband with feather, loincloth, brass bells.

   The American brought a new tactic that stunned the veteran English runners. He burst out at top speed, put in repeated surges, actually racing the entire event. Like their Redcoat ancestors at Lexington a century before, the local runners couldn't cope with this new, aggressive strategy. Deerfoot was rapidly crowned champion of England, and in 1863, he set a record for the one-hour run that stood for 34 years.

Have an Interesting Name

The 1898 Boston Marathon was won by Ronald McDonald (I kid you not). A 22-year-old Boston College student, he had never run a marathon before. But he had a pacing strategy. He held back 2 or 3 miles (3-5 km) behind the leaders until, reaching Wellesley at about the halfway point, he suddenly seemed to shift gears. Almost sprinting as he approached the finish, he passed "Ham" Gray, who was walking by this time, and crossed the line with a winning margin of three minutes. Ronald purportedly drank no fluids during the entire race.

Watch Where You're Going

Two years before Ronald McDonald's victory in Boston, 25 competitors ran the marathon event (24.9 miles) in the first of the modern Olympic Games in Athens. The Frenchman Albin Lermusiaux tried a strategy of blasting out with a blistering pace, and by the 15-kilometer mark he held a 3-kilometer lead over his nearest opponents. At this point, however, he was struck and knocked to the ground by the bicycle ridden by his coach. Lermusiaux eventually got back into the race, but was never again a factor.

Pay Attention to Your Opponents

In the 1970s, marathon champion Bill Rodgers generally liked to go out fast (the days of holding back in the marathon were long past). To aid in his pacing, he became an astute observer of just how his competitors were doing in the race. Did they look strained? Sweating too much? Struggling to breathe? (This foreshadows Lance Armstrong's famous look back at Jan Ullrich while struggling up L'Alpe d'Huez in the 2001 Tour de France.) One of his tactics was to engage them in conversation. "Boston Billy" figured that if they could respond with a full sentence at a pace of five minutes per mile at the 15th mile, they were still doing okay.[12]

Develop the Right Personality

The legendary Oregon runner Steve Prefontaine was—at least outwardly—brash, outspoken, confident, energetic, in your face. And he ran the same way. Always challenging, never holding back or giving up an inch. "Pre" wouldn't dream of sitting back and kicking at the end. He always tried to lead from the front, putting everything he had into every race. "A lot of people run a race to see who's the fastest," he once said. "I run to see who has the most guts."

It worked for him. In 1971, he had run 21 straight meets without a loss. By his freshman year at Oregon, he was on the cover of *Sports Illustrated*. During his brief career, which ended at the age of 24 in an automobile accident, he set American records for 2K, 3K (three times), 5K (four times), and 10K races.[2]

Keep an Eye on the clock

If ever there was an athlete who was a slave to time, it was the great Finnish runner Paavo Nurmi. Nurmi's achievements, which included 25 world records and 9 Olympic gold medals (in distances from 1,500 to 20,000 meters), have caused some to consider him the greatest distance runner in history. He's also the only runner to ever have an asteroid named after him (*1740 Paavo Nurmi*, identified by the Finnish astronomer Yrjö Väisälä in 1939).

Nurmi's philosophy during racing was to focus entirely on the clock. If he could pace himself to his goal time for distance, the opponents didn't matter. They'd fall to the wayside. To accomplish this, he always ran with a stopwatch in his hand, repeatedly consulting his split times, which he usually constructed to maintain an even pace. Sometimes, though, if he was enough in the lead, he'd toss the watch onto the infield in the final lap.

Much has been made of Nurmi's dark and withdrawn personality, quite the opposite of Steve Prefontaine's. He was an intense, obsessive, unfriendly person who was totally dedicated only to running. There is a story that when a statue of him running, completely lacking clothing, was unveiled in his birth city of Turku, Nurmi could only say, "I don't run naked."

Don't Let Them See You Sweat

And, finally, from the realm of literature comes the advice from Smith, the protagonist of *The Loneliness of the Long Distance Runner*, to "never let any of the other runners know you are in a hurry, even if you are. You can always overtake on long-distance running without letting the others smell the hurry in you."

These strategies for success notwithstanding, perhaps the best final advice comes from Carl Foster, who concluded that defining an optimal pacing strategy for a particular athlete in competitions of a specific distance, terrain, weather, and training status might be best considered a learning process.

Notes

1. Bannister, Roger. 1954. "The carbon dioxide stimulus to breathing in severe exercise." *Journal of Physiology* 125: 90-117. If you wish to be quite astounded by the level of Roger Bannister's physiology research, read this report. You probably won't understand much of it, but it will give you an appreciation of just how sophisticated Bannister's scientific knowledge of exercise physiology was. Bascomb, Neal. 2004. *The perfect mile*. New York: Mariner Books. Many excellent books have been written about Roger Bannister and his assault on the four-minute mile. This one is particularly exciting to read.

2. The latter provides a nice review of pacing strategies: Abbiss, Chris, and Paul Laursen. 2008. "Describing and understanding pacing strategies during athletic competition." *Sports Medicine* 38: 239-252. Foster, Carl et al. 1994. "Pacing strategy and athletic performance." *Sports Medicine* 17: 77-85.

3. Jordan, Tom. 1977. *Pre. The story of America's greatest running legend*. 2nd ed. Emmaus, PA: Rodale Press. Some, particularly European readers, may not recognize the name. Steve Prefontaine was popular, aggressive, cocky, and blessed with extraordinary distance-running talent. As Alberto Salazar said, "he made running cool." His life was tragically cut short by an automobile accident in 1975, when he was 24 years old. The fascinating details of his life can be found in this book.

4. "Deception" studies in pacing include: Albertus, Y. et al. 2005. "Effect of distance feedback on pacing strategy and perceived exertion during cycling," *Medicine and Science in Sports and Exercise* 37: 461-468; Morton, R.H 2009. "Deception by manipulating the clock calibration influence cycle ergometer endurance time in males," *Journal of Science and Medicine in Sport* 12: 332-337.

5. Readings on the central governor hypothesis include the following: Hill, A.V. et al. 1924. "Muscular exercise, lactic acid, and the supply and utilization of oxygen." *Proceedings of the Royal Society of Britain* 97: 438-475. Kayser, B. 2003. "Exercise starts and ends in the brain." *European Journal of Applied Physiology* 90: 411-419. Lambert, E.V. et al. 2005. "Complex systems model of fatigue: Integrative homeostatic control of peripheral physiological systems during exercise in humans." *British Journal of Sports Medicine* 39: 52-62. Noakes, T.D. et al. 2004. "From catastrophe to complexity: A novel model of integrative central neural regulation of effort and fatigue during exercise in humans." *British Journal of Sports Medicine* 38: 511-514. Shephard, R. 2009. "Is it time to retire the central governor?" *Sports Medicine* 39: 709-721.

6. Information on top-down brain functioning can be found in the following article: Engel, A.K. et al. 2001. "Dynamic predictions: Oscillations and synchrony in top-down processing." *Nature Reviews* 2: 704-716.

7. For a discussion of heatstroke and marathon running, see the following: Rae, D.E. et al. 2008. "Heatstroke during endurance exercise: Is there evidence for excessive endothermy?" *Medicine and Science in Sports and Exercise* 40: 1193-1204. Roberts, W.O. 2005. "Common threads in a random tapestry. Another viewpoint on exertional heatstroke." *The Physician and Sports Medicine* 33: 42-49.

8. Read more about cycling all-out strategies in this article: Aisbett, B., P. Lerossignol, G.K. McConnell, C.R. Abbiss., and R. Snow. 2009. "Influence of all-out and fast start on 5-min cycling time trial performance." *Medicine and Science in Sports and Exercise* 41: 1965-1971.

9. The unexplained pacing strategy insisted upon by competitive rowers is discussed in the following article: Garland, S.W. 2005. "An analysis of the pacing strategy adopted by elite competitors in 200-m rowing." *British Journal of Sports Medicine* 39: 39-42.

10. One, of course, is the backstroke in swimming. The other, not so obvious, is the tug-of-war. Not a real sport, you say? Pish! You're obviously unaware of the Tug-of-War International Federation (TWIF), a 47-year-old organization with 25 member countries that conducts annual regional and world championships. In fact, the tug-of-war was included in the Olympic Games until 1920. Now you know.

11. References for these research studies include the following: Foster et al. 1993. "Physiological responses during simulated competition." *Medicine and Science in Sports and Exercise* 25: 877-882. Gosztyla, A.E. et al. 2006. "The impact of different pacing strategies on five-kilometer running time trial performance." *Journal of Strength and Conditioning Research* 20: 882-886. Hettinga, F.J. et al. 2007. "Biodynamics. Effect of pacing strategy on energy expenditure during a 1500-m cycling time trial." *Medicine and Science in Sports and Exercise* 39: 2212-2218. Robinson, S. 1958. "Influence of fatigue on the efficiency of men during exhaustive runs." *Journal of Applied Physiology* 12: 197-201. Thompson, K.G. et al. 2003. "The effect of even, positive, and negative pacing on metabolic, kinematic, and temporal variables during breast stroke swimming." *European Journal of Applied Physiology* 88: 438-443.

12. Derderian, Tom. 1994. *Boston Marathon. The history of the world's premier running event.* Champaign, IL: Human Kinetics. Krise, Raymond, and Bill Squires. 1982. *Fast tracks. The history of distance running.* Brattleboro, VT: The Stephen Greene Press. Information on Deerfoot, Ronald McDonald, and other early heroes of running are nicely presented in these books.

TAKE-HOME MESSAGES

1. Traditionally, selecting a speed during a distance running, cycling, or swimming race has been considered to be under the control of the athlete, who selects a best pace based on physical sensations of the level of fatigue. More recently, however, it has been suggested that an unconscious governor within the brain sets the pace (based on previous racing experience) as a way of protecting the athlete from potential damaging effects.

2. In their quest to go beyond the pain, athletes need to heed the wisdom of such signals of fatigue, particularly in race conditions with high temperatures or humidity.

3. Optimal pacing strategy during a distance event for an individual athlete is probably best determined by trial and error.

4. Although small positive or negative deviations (less than 2%) at the start are allowable, most advise keeping a near-steady pace throughout.

5. The tortoise had it right. Avoid jackrabbit starts.

CHAPTER 2

This chapter takes up where the last one ended. We have (or our subconscious brain has) decided on an optimal pacing strategy for our distance race—the optimal means of expending energy (regulating speed) relative to time to provide the best performance result. Now, how are we going to go about doing this? We will hand this task over to an automatic motor oscillator within the central nervous system, one which has the wisdom to decide for runners how best to turn their legs over with time (stride frequency) and to determine the length of their stride. For swimmers, cyclists, and rowers, it's probably the same story. The nature and even the location of this subconscious motor controller—driven by an internal clock—remains mysterious. But it seems most likely that athletes had best adhere to its decisions.

MARCHING TO THE SAME DRUMMER

Cadence in Endurance Events

Normally, the cockroach, that repugnant six-legged creature, that pariah of refined persons everywhere, moves himself about in a rather peculiar manner. He balances on three legs (the front and back on one side, the middle one on the other). Then he pushes off and switches to the other three. The cockroach wanders around your kitchen floor at night, as it were, like an alternating tripod.

But put him in a race, and suddenly everything changes. He shifts his weight backward and scurries about with incredible alacrity on just the two back legs, a bipedal locomotion that almost mimics upright runners like you and me. If you have a desire to watch this, you can fly any January 26th to the Story Bridge Hotel in Brisbane, where they celebrate the national holiday (Australia Day) by hosting the World Championship Cockroach Races. This event, which draws many hundreds of rowdies and is accompanied by live bands, TV coverage, and heavy betting (not to mention a little beer), has been going on annually since 1982. It's where you stack your animal, who scurries to the finish in a boxing-style ring, against the best in the country. It's the Super Bowl, the Final Four, the World Series of cockroach racing.

How does the cockroach accomplish this magical feat of locomotion? What, physiologically speaking, wins the race? Well, within that minuscule nervous system of his, the victor possesses an altogether highly talented control center. And, with the aid of what must be a very tiny timekeeping clock, it signals his legs to move in a coordinated, alternative fashion. Add to this another master clock in the brain that sets the tempo of the whole motor machine. It's an extraordinarily complex mechanism, to be sure.

Now this may come as a bit of abhorrent news, but you and this lowly pest actually share these same masterful neurological devices, the controllers that command how we run, bike, and swim. That's right. The same ones. Read on.

The Beat Goes On: The Motor Controller

Consider for a moment the dragon boat. In this narrow craft, 20 paddlers sit facing forward, side by side, competing at distances of 200 to 2,000 meters. Although dragon boat racing is currently experiencing a burst of international popularity, in fact, it has a very ancient history, dating to Chinese water festivals more than 2,500 years ago. The boats are a great deal of fun to watch, with their decorative Chinese dragon heads and tails (figure 2.1). If you head off to Queens, New York, in August, you can witness one of the biggest dragon boat festivals in the United States, with more than 145 teams competing.

At the front of the boat, facing backward, sits the drummer, who signals the stroke cadence to the paddlers by the rhythmic beating of a large drum as the boat surges through the water. Bam! Bam! Bam! The sound echoes down the river as the drummer beats out the indicated pace. Given environmental conditions, the boat's proximity to the finish line and position relative to other boats, the drummer alters the tempo, thereby affecting the work of the paddlers, all the while maintaining a beautifully coordinated synchronization of effort.

The drummer, I feel confident in saying, would never consider himself an intrinsic motor oscillator, but that's exactly what he is. With his rhythmic beating, he directs the tempo of a complex motor system (the 20 paddlers) that drives the boat forward. In each of us,

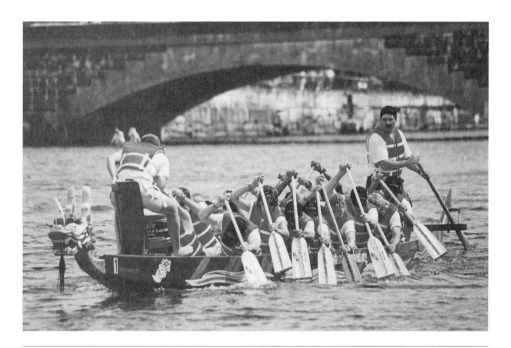

FIGURE 2.1. A dragon boat heads down river to the drum's resounding tempo.
Will Wang, Hong Kong Dragon Boat Festival of Boston, 2004.

too, there exists a sort of dragon boat drummer, an automatic motor controller residing somewhere in our central nervous system that coordinates the many parts of the motor's machinery and regulates the tempo at which they should turn over.

Just as dragon boat drummers rely on their sense of rhythm to maintain a regular cadence, so our intrinsic controllers of muscular activity listen to an internal clock that, like a metronome, keeps a steady tempo of neuromuscular activation.

Our central motor oscillator is highly intelligent, able to select for the distance runner, for example, an optimal combination of stride frequency and stride length that is most energy efficient for optimizing performance. It's a controller that, left unperturbed, is amazingly stable. And, best of all, it does this all without causing us to think about it.

Caution! Don't confuse this central motor oscillator with the alleged central governor we encountered in the previous chapter. Their names are similar, but they're altogether different directors. They work out of different cubicles, even on separate floors. We all possess the former, which controls the pattern and rate of muscle contractions that let us walk, run, swim, and cycle. The other is a proposed strategizer (with a brake) that might determine our pace during racing and could keep us from dangerous levels of overexertion.

In this chapter, we're going to explore the characteristics of this automatic motor oscillator. We'll examine the means by which it decides the best pattern of muscular activity per unit time. To use runners as an example, it deduces which is the right combination of stride frequency and stride length to attain a desired velocity. And, we'll look at some recent research that has tried to decipher the location and nature of this central oscillator, both in humans and animals. We'll start out using a model of distance running, since most research has involved this type of locomotion. Then we'll add on what is known about selecting best cadences for other events, such as swimming, cycling, and rowing.

The overriding practical question here is can athletes manipulate their stride frequency, pedaling rate, or stroke rate as they strategize for best performance? If so, should they? Or, should they rely on the wisdom of the body's subconscious, timekeeping clocks, which have developed through hundreds of thousands of centuries of biological evolution?

Muscular Coordination: Stride Frequency and Length

Bang! The 10K starting gun fires and the rhythmic cycle of neuromuscular events begins. The hip joint flexes (during the swing phase when the foot is in the air), then extends (with the foot in contact with the ground during the support phase). Similar alternations occur at the knee and ankle. The muscular activity generating these joint displacements is highly stereotyped. At the initial foot touchdown, the hip and knee joint extensors are activated (gluteus maximus, gastrocnemius). The vastus lateralis and vastus medialis muscles of the thigh become active at the beginning of the support phase. The semitendinosus and semimembranosus, hip extensors and knee flexors, contract at the end of the swing phase and continue during the support phase. Meanwhile, the ankle is acted on by the gastrocnemius (plantar flexion) and the tibialis anterior (dorsiflexion).

So far, so good. You've just taken one step! Now the motor oscillator orchestrating all this begins to fire with unrelenting automatism in clocklike fashion, repeating this succession of finely coordinated muscular contractions the many thousands of times required to deliver you to the finish line, all the while keeping you from landing on your nose. Again, you can be grateful this all occurs at an unconscious level.

According to chapter 1, the motor oscillator has received information about the amount of muscular work per time (velocity) that will predict optimal performance for the distance and conditions of that particular race, either from you (by cognitive pacing strategies), a central governor, or both. Now, besides simply coordinating the synchronization of all these muscle groups, the oscillator has an additional task—figuring out the best means of producing the desired velocity. In doing so, it has two choices. It can elect to manipulate the firing rate of the automatic controller (increase the stride frequency—the drummer in the dragon boat would bang faster to increase the cadence of the paddlers and the speed of the dragon boat). Or (this is something the dragon boat drummer can't do), it can alter the length of each stride by adjusting the mechanics and force of muscular contraction. How does it decide which to do? More strides or longer strides per time? At first glance, it would seem hypothetically possible, at least within physical constraints, to utilize either mechanism to adjust race velocity. But, as the next section shows, that isn't true. But why should one mechanism be preferable to the other?

Empirical Observations

If you were sitting next to Jack Daniels high in the stands at the 1984 Olympic Games, you certainly would have wondered what on earth this man was doing. Well, he was counting. In fact, so was his wife Nancy. They were recording the number of times that runners turned over their legs—their stride frequency—during events ranging from 800 meters to the marathon. Daniels was—and still is—a scientist and coach driven by an insatiable curiosity. (He and fellow physiologist Gary Krahenbuhl once designed a pair of Styrofoam shoes that enabled them to walk on water—successfully, it turned out—across the width of Dr. Krahenbuhl's backyard swimming pool). In the Los Angeles Games, he was trying to figure out how successful athletes varied their stride length and frequency during competitions. What he found was very interesting. For events ranging in length from 3,000 meters to the marathon, almost all the runners had the same stride frequency (a cadence of around 180 steps per minute, or 90 steps with each foot). When they picked up the pace in each of these events, they did so by increasing their stride length. The stride frequency stayed the same. (In the shorter races, the stride frequency was somewhat faster.)

In his coaching experience, Daniels has found that inexperienced runners often have a slower cadence. He thinks this practice wastes energy and can lead to injuries, since slow stride frequencies launch the body into the air longer, causing greater impact on landing. He tells his runners to go lightly while getting into a rhythm of 180 steps per minute. "Imagine that you're running over a field of raw eggs," he says, "and you don't want to break any of them."

The findings are much the same when subjects are taken into the exercise testing laboratory. Peter Cavanagh and Rodger Kram at Penn State University measured stride frequency and length in a group of 18- to 40-year-old distance runners at treadmill speeds between 3 and 4 meters per second. These speeds are equivalent to a range of race speeds between 8:58 and 6:44 minutes per mile, which they considered typical of recreational runners. Interestingly, between these speeds, increases in treadmill velocity (33%) were paralleled by a similar increase in stride length (28%), but little change was observed in stride frequency (up 6%). That is, as running velocity rose through this range of real-world distance racing speeds, stride frequency remained relatively constant. As the subjects ran faster, they relied more on extending stride length.[1]

In another study, patterns of stride frequency and stride length for the top finishers in the 1,500-meter, 5,000-meter, and 10,000-meter events were observed in an elite-level international meet. Race velocities for these events averaged approximately 6.3, 5.7, and 5.5 meters per second, respectively. Top finishers in the 1,500-meter race had a stride length 12% longer and a stride frequency 2% greater than those in the 10K race. So, again we see evidence that within the velocity range of distance running competition, changes in speed were achieved predominantly by altering stride length, rather than stride frequency.

So, you've just passed the 4-mile (6 km) mark of a 10K road race, and, surprisingly, you really feel pretty darn good. Time to turn up the pace! You tell your hard-working motor controller to go faster. It responds by increasing your stride length, leaving the tempo (or the firing rate) of the oscillator pretty much unchanged.

Explaining the Constant Tempo

The alert reader should now be ready with the next question: For distance runners, why is stride frequency—how fast the legs turn over—so relatively constant at different speeds? What keeps the motor oscillator firing at pretty much the same tempo as they move up their running speeds? What are the biological advantages? And is there a price to pay if runners try to manipulate stride frequency and stride length on their own? Let's consider some possible answers to these questions.

Experience has taught exercise scientists that when confronted with questions of why body systems function the way they do, that the answer usually lies in the most efficient expenditure of energy. We are constantly reminded that biological systems are devised so as to perform most economically, with minimal expenditure of metabolic energy. From a Darwinian perspective, this makes sense. The less energy (read *food stores*) required to perform life's activities, the greater the survival value. It would be reasonable to assume that the best stride frequency (SF), stride length (SL), or ratio of SF to SL, might have been selected in the process of evolution, with the goal of minimizing energy cost during locomotion or optimizing work efficiency. Experimental evidence bears this out.

If you ask subjects to run on a treadmill at a constant speed, say 5 miles (8 km) per hour, you can determine their energy expenditure by measuring how much oxygen their bodies use (oxygen uptake, or $\dot{V}O_2$). Now, keep the treadmill speed the same, but have them run at several different combinations of stride length and frequency. If you plot a graph of $\dot{V}O_2$ versus either of these, you will see a U-shaped curve, as indicated in figure 2.2. Obviously, a particular tempo of the motor controller (a certain stride frequency that matches the lowest energy demand) is most economical for these particular runners. And if the subjects deviate from this rate or stride length, the energy cost goes up.

The fascinating part of this is that now, if you simply ask the subjects to run at a speed that they prefer, it almost always nearly coincides with that most economical velocity. That central motor oscillator has keen insight. It knows what speed will cost runners the least metabolic work, dictating this without even consulting them.[2]

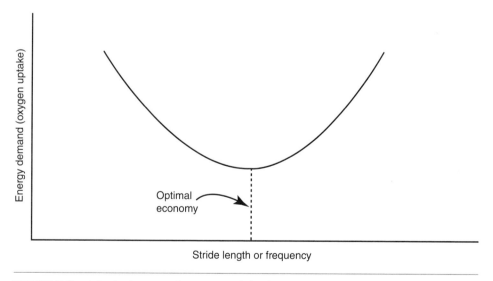

FIGURE 2.2. A typical curve of oxygen uptake (energy demand) plotted against stride length or frequency when a subject is running at identical speeds. The nadir of the curve represents the stride length or frequency with the greatest energy economy.

The next question, of course, is why does metabolic demand change as you alter the speed and stride length? What is so special about the selected cadence that makes it the most economical in terms of energy? The answer must lie in the complex tangle of biomechanical factors that accompany locomotion. Such a discussion clearly lies beyond the scope of this chapter, but here are a few of the likely suspects.

1. As runners turn up the stride frequency, their muscles are called upon to contract at a faster velocity. The energy required for a muscle to contract is directly related to the speed of its contraction. Thus, increasing running cadence does not economize energy. And it costs more to increase the frequency than to increase the stride length as the subjects run faster.

2. In this equation, you must consider that propulsion with running is not simply the consequence of leg-muscle contraction. The act of running can be considered a series of forward jumps, with the elasticity of nonmuscular structures, such as tendons and ligaments, contributing significantly to the work. And that rebound helps minimize energy costs. Running has been likened to a mass bouncing along on springs. This propulsive effect is more than minor. The stride length, not the frequency, benefits from the energy savings. It has been suggested that while running at middle-distance speeds, the work required to propel the body forward is achieved half by muscular forces and half by elastic recoil.

3. The motor oscillator remains quite stable during steady-state locomotion, but a certain small stride-to-stride change over time still exists in the cadence. If you plot the amount of this variability against stride frequency, you see that U-shaped curve where a certain cadence is associated with the lowest variability. Interestingly, in studies of subjects walking, this frequency of minimizing variability matches up with that of the greatest energy economy.[3]

4. When stride frequency is increased, of course, the number of times the foot strikes the ground in a minute increases. In contrast, the time the foot actually makes contact with ground during each stride is shortened. The force necessary to move the body weight against gravity for each stride, however, remains constant. That means that the rate of force the foot must apply to the ground for each stride goes up as stride frequency is increased. The implication might be, then, that the risk of stress injury to the leg is increased by greater stride rates.

So, what does all this tell us about selecting stride frequency during distance-running competitions? Let's go back to the runners who want to pick up the pace at the 4-mile mark. What would happen if they increase their race speed at this point by turning over their legs faster, purposefully overriding the natural tempo of the motor oscillator and increasing stride frequency? If you are impressed with the research data described in the preceding section, you might expect that they might, at least temporarily, increase their race speed. However, the price of this choice is exaggerated energy demand and musculoskeletal stress. So, in addition to increasing risk of overuse injury, performance might well be compromised.

On the other hand, notes the skeptic, you do not hear nightmare stories of running catastrophes resulting from pushing stride frequency during distance racing. How these findings actually might (or might not) translate into performance outcomes has never, to my knowledge, been tested. Too, the question has been raised that the magnitude of the negative effects of self-generated cadence might not be appreciable. From their studies, Peter Cavanagh and Keith Williams contended that selection of an optimal ratio between stride length and frequency is not a major determinant of running economy for trained distance runners. Instead, they note, factors such as biomechanical parameters (smoothness of gait, contributions of elastic recoil, and footwear) are much more likely to play important roles in energy economy during running.[4]

For my money, I'll stick to the opinion of most running coaches that you had best leave the selection of stride frequency and length to the wisdom of the central motor generator, whose thousands of years of experience probably outweigh that of a 25-year-old upstart. To paraphrase the old margarine advertisement, it's not a good idea to mess with Mother Nature. There is actually some solid science behind the idea that stride frequency and length adopted during competition by an individual runner in a given race are automatically selected for a good reason. Energy demands are minimized and conscious efforts to perturb either stride frequency or stride length are probably counterproductive for optimal performance. Here's the bottom line: Distance runners should not be too quick to cognitively manipulate stride frequency and length during competition. Instead, they should stick to those that come naturally.

One way to avoid deviating from instinct is to mentally dissociate during running—that is, think about anything other than the immediacy of the race. Divert your thoughts to what you're having for dinner that night or your plans for the summer. (If the race is a long one, you could review your entire senior year in high school.) In other words, go on autopilot and let your unconscious regulators in the brain do their job. You might shut out some of the discomfort of the running competition. You also won't interfere with the optimal stride frequency and stride length settings at a given velocity that are prescribed by the controller in your central nervous system.

It's interesting that when Bill Morgan studied this phenomenon, he found that average middle-of-the-pack marathon runners tended to do just that. They kept their minds on something other than the race itself. Runners at a more elite level were actually more likely to control their behavior during a race. They closely monitored how they felt, the mechanics of their stride, the distance covered, and so on. Just what this means in terms of allowing the brain to keep the best running mechanics is not altogether clear.[5]

Cadence and Other Sports

So much for running. Let's see what we know about optimal stroke rates in other sports, most particularly those that are not weight bearing in nature.

Swimming

We now move from bipedal locomotion against the forces of gravity to arm motion versus the resistance of water—very different forms of exercise. But there are many parallels in the story of optimization of stroke rates in distance swimmers and stride frequency of runners, with a few twists in the plot.

Mathematically, it's the same issue. The number of arm strokes in the water multiplied by the distance traveled per stroke equals the velocity. The former is determined by the tempo of the motor oscillator and is characteristically an energy-expensive means of generating speed. The latter, more energy efficient, is created by factors such as the power of the stroke, drag reduced by body position, leg force while kicking, and hand size. The swimmer will move through the water at the highest velocity for any particular distance with a particular combination of stroke rate and stroke distance. Finding that optimal ratio for a particular athlete in a given event is a critical component of swim training. The extent to which this best ratio of stroke frequency to distance reflects an intrinsic pacemaker, with knowledge of factors like work efficiency and minimizing energy demands, is unclear. As a corollary, then, it is controversial whether swimmers should be taught to manipulate stroke rates or to leave them to their intuition.

That's the summary. Let's back up now and examine the details. If you have swimmers perform a series of maximal distance swims and then plot their velocity versus different stroke rates, you'll see the same inverted U-shaped curve we saw for runners. There's a best stroke rate, and it corresponds to the one that the swimmer prefers. This sounds a lot like a central controller subconsciously dictating an individual swimmer's optimal ratio of stroke rate to distance, much like we considered for distance running.

In general, differences in velocity in the performance of swimmers at the elite level have been attributed to variations in distance per stroke, not stroke rate. In fact, the stroke rate that allows swimmers to achieve their maximal velocity is often similar. A comparison of the times in the U.S. Olympic swimming trials between 1976 and 1984 found that the average velocity was greater in 1984 in 9 out of 10 women's events and in 3 of the 10 men's events. Of these 12 improvements, the increased velocity was accounted for by a 4 to 16% increase in stroke distance. In 8 of these, there was a concomitant fall in stroke rate (a loss of 3 to 13%). The increased race speed was due exclusively to faster stroke rates in only two short events (women's 100-meter butterfly and 100-meter backstroke).

When fatigue and slowing of velocity occur near the end of a distance swim race, it is almost always due to a decrease in distance per stroke. Presumably, this reflects a diminishing ability to generate force to overcome water resistance (that is, a decline in production of muscle power), but other issues might be involved, such as increased drag from poor body alignment as the swimmer tires. Interestingly, a number of observers have found that swimmers often increase their stroke rate near the end of a race in an attempt to compensate for this decline in stroke distance as fatigue sets in.

The best way for a swimmer to increase race velocity, then, would be to train to increase muscle power to propel the body, to learn to carve out an effective stroke pattern, and to assume and maintain a proper, hydrodynamic body position in the water. For most swimmers, training to increase velocity over distance by increasing stroke rate is not expected to be beneficial, since it only shortens the stroke length. Most people find that the tempo of the central motor oscillator does not like to be perturbed.

The preceding information describes trends of stroke rate and distance seen in competitive distance swimmers. But it is important to realize that if you sit by the pool and watch top competitors, you will, in fact, see all sorts of combinations of stroke length and distance for achieving race speed. Some elite swimmers have found success with high stroke rates, others with low. Some increase speed by turning over the arms faster, others by a more powerful stroke. Some show a falloff in both stroke frequency and length as fatigue sets in. In others, stroke rate progressively declines as the race progresses.[6]

In this mélange of styles and preferences, it is difficult to sort out the role that an intrinsic motor oscillator might have in selecting, below the level of consciousness, the ratio of stroke frequency to length that would be the most energy efficient. For coaches and athletes, this boils down to a long-standing controversy: Should swimmers be taught to train and compete at a certain stroke frequency and length? Or, should they go with what feels intuitively right (which would be saying that the message on proper stroke frequency comes from a subconscious, intrinsic timekeeper)? There is no agreement on the question.

David Pendergast is an exercise physiologist at the State University of New York at Buffalo who has devoted his career to understanding the factors that go into successful swimming. He notes that "it is known that swimmers left to self-select a frequency: velocity ratio will swim at a stroke frequency that results in less than their maximal velocity. However, whether this frequency can be sustained for given distances remains an issue. One must consider 'what feels right' may also be influenced by the swimmer's training. That is, training at lower velocity and frequency may make swimming at higher velocities and stroke rates uncomfortable."

But, all this uncertainty notwithstanding, there is one concrete strategy here. Don't fret over whether a subconscious central governor is in charge or not, just experiment! Do a few time trials while varying stroke frequency, and see what happens to the finish time. The goal would be to find the slowest stroke cadence that still maintains a top velocity.

The veteran coach E.W. Maglischo summed it up this way. "One job of the coach is to help athletes find the optimum combination of stroke rate and length that will allow them to swim at some desired speed with the least energy expenditure. That combination will undoubtedly be different for each swimmer and each event. There is no guarantee that swimmers self-select the best combination of stroke rate and stroke length."[6]

Important, too, is the idea that the best combination of stroke frequency and length at the beginning of the race, in a rested condition, is probably going to be very different from that near the end of the event, when the swimmer faces increased levels of fatigue. So, experimenting to find how a particular swimmer should strategize an optimal ratio of rate to length during competition should be done in both conditions.

Knowing your best stroke frequency may come in handy. Suppose you dive into the pool trying for a gold medal in the 200-meter butterfly. Suddenly, you're blinded—your goggles have filled with water. That's what happened to Michael Phelps during the Beijing Olympic Games. No problem! Unable to see his opponents or the oncoming wall, he simply counted his well-tuned strokes to estimate when to make his turns. The result? A world record time of 1:52.03. You should be so lucky.

Cycling

On the wall of my study hangs a print of Pierre and Marie Curie. They're standing in front of their Paris home in 1894, ready to take a ride on the new bicycles they gave each other as wedding gifts. The cost of about 200 francs each must have made the bikes quite an extravagance (Pierre's annual salary was 3,600 francs). Marie looks happy, but she's wearing a look of quiet determination. This is perhaps just some leftover fatigue from all those hours of mixing pitchblende in the laboratory. I find this photo captivating. In one image, we see the joy of living, of devoted human relationships, of exercise, of the rewards of committed scientific work. And it reminds us that scientists and bicycles have never been too far apart.

During that latter part of the 19th century, the popularity of the bicycle was spreading rapidly. Inevitably, so was bicycle racing. In 1903, to promote the circulation of his newspaper, Henri Desgrange devised a six-day event he called "le Tour de France," which drew 60 entrants for a 2,397-km race throughout the French countryside. (It worked. The circulation of *L'Auto* doubled by the race date.) It was apparent to scientists watching these competitors struggle through this grueling competition that cyclists were like machines—you fed them fuel, and they converted energy to mechanical work, like unconscious automatons. You could, evidently, readily study this human motor in the laboratory and gain an understanding of which factors determined cycling performance.

Furthermore, it was expected that such scientific research should be able to provide practical information that would be useful for cyclists in learning the best means of training and competing. Thus began a long marriage between science and cycling, one that today has brought us lightweight machines, ways of reducing wind resistance, proper diets, and heart rate monitors.

As information from such research began to unfold, one observation noted early on that still sticks with us today has proven perplexing. It is not at all well explained. By now, you are quite familiar with the supposition that from many different perspectives, conservation of energy is a key element to success in distance sports. If energy supply is a central determinant of athletic performance in terms of aerobic endurance, we would expect that the minimum energy expenditure for any level of athletic work would be advantageous. That is, the greatest amount of work (power output in running, swimming, rowing, or cycling) that you can do with the least amount of energy (higher work efficiency), the longer you should be able to exercise at a given velocity, or the higher the speed you should be able to achieve for a given distance.

We've already seen much evidence for this in these pages. In walking, running, and probably swimming, the preferred cadence (selected by the athlete) is the one that is usually the most economical energetically, and is associated with the greatest velocity.

It's a neat conceptual package, and we like it because it makes sense.

But then we come to cycling. If you take different pedaling rates while the subject is performing the same amount of work, and then plot these values against metabolic demand (oxygen uptake), you see, like with running, a particular pedaling cadence that is best, that is the most energy efficient. And that cadence has been repeatedly shown to be around 50 to 60 revolutions per minute (rpm). Moreover, the same rate of pedaling has been linked to optimal levels of other markers of metabolic stress, such as heart rate, muscle production of lactic acid, and lung ventilation. Fair enough, but what is difficult to understand is that competitive cyclists normally pedal at frequencies of 90 to 105 rpm, almost twice as fast. According to what we know, this should be terribly energy inefficient, a real detriment to successful performance.

Alejandro Lucia and his fellow Spanish investigators nicely demonstrated this when they recorded pedaling rates of elite cyclists competing in the Tour de France, Giro d'Italia, and the Vuelta a España. The average cadence was 71 rpm during uphill cycling (through the high mountain passes), 92 rpm for individual time trials, and 89 rpm during flat, long stages. Pedaling rates rose to about 110 rpm for brief periods of accelerations or breakaways. Studies indicate that if you increase the pedaling cadence by 60 to 100% (from around 50 to 90 rpm), while keeping the work output constant, you'll increase energy cost by 14 to 21%. That's a very appreciable amount of energy. Think about that when you power your way up Mt. Ventoux during your next Tour de France.

It's not just elite cyclists who pedal at these fast, energy-efficient cadences. Anthony Marsh and Philip Martin compared the effect of changing cadence on metabolic demand and the preferred cadence of eight trained cyclists and eight untrained subjects. They all cycled at the same work load of 200 watts.

The most energy-efficient cadence (lowest $\dot{V}O_2$) was 56 rpm for the cyclists and 63 rpm for the untrained subjects. But the preferred cadence was 85 rpm and 92 rpm for the two groups, respectively. In this particular study, the difference between oxygen demand at the most efficient and preferred cadence was not very great, about 5%.

Why does the motor oscillator of the world's best cyclists (and even you and me) fire at this extraordinarily high tempo that is apparently energy inefficient? Many think it has something to do with minimizing muscle strain. At a fixed work load, the faster you pedal, the less the force on the pedals per revolution. That would seem to make sense. You would suppose, then, that the rating of perceived exertion (RPE)—how the cyclist feels—would be lowest at those 80- to 100-rpm cadences, Alas, not so. In fact, investigations of RPE at various pedaling rates have provided very inconsistent results. Some have verified a minimum RPE at a cadence of 80 to 100 rpm, others have found a nadir of RPE at 60 to 70 rpm. In the preceding study by Marsh and Martin, RPE was pretty flat between 65 and 80 rpm, but then increased at faster pedaling rates. Their conclusion? "RPE may not be a critical variable in cadenced selection during submaximal power output cycling."[7]

So, just why an intrinsic pacer insists on pedaling at a high cadence during cycling remains a mystery. Is it a trade-off between minimizing muscle strain (best at high cadences) and maximizing energy efficiency of muscles (best at low cadences)? Sometimes, perhaps when more than one factor creates a best cadence, even the intrinsic motor oscillator has to make compromises. Perhaps, too, the controller of tempo is listening to physiological or mechanical messages that, to cite the Bard, are more than are dreamt of in our philosophy.

Maybe that philosophy has something to do with the function of the skeletal muscle as an auxiliary circulatory pump. This is an idea that been around for a long time in scientific circles, although it has been difficult to study and confirm. But many are in agreement that as the skeletal muscles contract around veins, they create a pumping action that propels blood flow, much as the heart does. The downside of this is that as the muscles contract at high levels of force, they actually close off the blood vessels and impede, rather than promote, blood flow.

During cycling, pedal cadence may have something to do with this. Researchers at Colorado State University showed that as cadence was increased from 70 to 110 rpm (keeping the work load constant), the output of the heart increased. That rise was in excess of increases in metabolic rate. These authors concluded that the skeletal muscle pumped blood more effectively at high cadences. This fits, since such rapid pedaling rates are associated with less force per revolution. Consequently, the veins in the muscle would be less occluded and blood flow would be more free.[8]

And, finally, a couple of other ideas spring to mind as to why cycling may be an anomaly in this question of cadence and economy. First, because the bicycle is a machine, maybe it operates outside of evolutionary forces that have influenced human muscle function. And, second, perhaps the explanation is somewhere in the fact that a bicycle does not permit you to increase stride length, only cadence.

To Summarize....

In this chapter, we've encountered a pacemaker that orders the sequence of innervation of our limb muscles so we can run, swim, bike, and row. This oscillator originated as deeply in our evolutionary past as the process of animal locomotion. And then there's a separate subconscious motor oscillator that governs the ratio of frequency, tempo, or muscle activation to its force production while listening carefully to an intrinsic clock. It controls how frequently (at what rate) we contract our limb muscles. It controls our stride rate in running, our stroke rate during swimming and rowing, and our pedaling cadence when we cycle.

We can override the decisions of this second motor pacer by our conscious decisions. But there is evidence, at least for runners, that if left unperturbed, this controller will pick the tempo that is energetically best, the one that will optimize performance. If so, it will be counterproductive for the athlete to purposefully alter cadence in these sports beyond what feels natural. And so, going with what intuitively feels right generally seems to be the best advice.

Central Pattern Generator

Thus far, this chapter has discussed how a central motor oscillator might act, but it has ignored the more difficult and challenging question of what it is. How does it work? Where is it located? Can it be manipulated? So, it's time now to explore the nature of this metronomic central controller that coordinates our exercising machine, sets the tempo, and regulates muscular force, all below the level of our consciousness. Indeed, the oscillator doesn't even consult us in these matters, freeing us to dream of athletic glory.

In terms of any clear understanding of just how this central controller works, we're still pretty much in the dark. But the story of the timekeepers of motor performance—the internal clocks that tick away, governing locomotion and athletic success—is an intriguing one. One important point of this excursion into some basic science is that these timing mechanisms that operate beneath our awareness are coded in our genetic material and are the end product of hundreds of thousands of years of evolutionary time. We need to appreciate their extraordinary wisdom.

But first, some terminology. Let's be correct about this. Throughout the first portion of this chapter, I have taken liberties with the vocabulary, using all sorts of descriptive names for this central machine, such as *oscillator, controller,* or *regulator.* The official term utilized by card-carrying neurobiologists is *central pattern generator,* or CPG. So, that's what we'll use from now on.

Biological Nature of the CPG

If you think about it, all muscular activity in the body is characterized by rhythmicity. Peristaltic motion of the gut, beating of the heart, breathing, chewing, swallowing—they all rely on a central neurologic clock that controls rate (or tempo) and synchronizes sequence of muscular activity. Vital body functions depend on it, not just locomotion.

The basis of this idea of a CPG is that certain nerve cells located in the central nervous system (brain and spinal cord) can spontaneously and independently generate regular, clocklike electrical impulses. The timing and rate of these rhythmic electrical discharges is by some means signaled to those cells responsible for commanding the coordinated and repetitive contraction of skeletal muscle that permits locomotion. Indeed, such neurons within and outside the central nervous system with spontaneous oscillatory electrical properties are well known (the heart's pacemaker—the sinus node—is an obvious example). Understanding just how such single-cell electrical generators can be combined into systems that regulate the muscular complexities of running, swimming, and cycling remains, quite clearly, a large challenge.

This CPG is not just one central controller. A good analogy might be that it is a system of franchises, or a number of separate timepieces with different functions that coordinate and synchronize the exact sequence of muscular innervation over time that permits locomotion. If you run faster, that sequence of muscle contraction must necessarily be maintained by some timekeeper. Another clock precisely regulates the tempo of the entire system. If you want to kick to the finish, that clock speeds up with metronomic regularity. A host of additional controllers adjust coordination and balance in space, receive information from the periphery, and listen to your cognitive commands. Given the multitude of the functional components, it is not difficult to recognize, then, that the CPG is not a single wizard sitting at the controls in Oz, but rather several control centers that are dispersed throughout the central nervous system. Indeed, we can predict that the CPG is, in reality, a functional network. We'll keep that idea in mind as we examine the nature of the CPG in animals and humans a bit later.

A good deal of research interest currently exists about CPGs and how they work. Admittedly, how they relate to athletic performance has not been at the top of the priority list. Insights into the basic mechanisms of rhythmic motor movements have been of more interest. This research activity has been recently energized by more practical issues—the potential for rehabilitation of stroke patients and those with spinal cord injuries, for instance, or how to design propulsion mechanisms for robots.

Almost all insights into the existence, function, and location of CPGs have come from work with animals, particularly in studies looking at effects of surgical interruption of different portions of the nervous system. (Human subjects are traditionally resistant to dissection of the spinal cord.) Indeed, with a quick run through the literature, you can become enlightened on matters ranging from CPG control of intestinal activity in lobsters, to regulation of the heartbeat in leeches, to the initiation of vomiting of dogs. New information regarding CPGs is becoming available for humans, too. We will review this in the following section. All would suggest that the basic control of rhythmic motor activity in you and me is similar to that observed throughout the animal kingdom. This observation has supported an assumption that development of CPGs originates from the obscure evolutionary past, and that they have been critical to the growth of the evolutionary animal tree. More particularly, it also supports the likelihood that animal models can serve as appropriate surrogates for humans in investigations of CPGs.

One other point. It is obvious that CPGs, wherever they are located, must be influenced by brain structures that accept sensory information from the outside (for example, cats dash out of the way as they see a car approaching) and, in humans, cognitive decision making (I want to run faster). However, CPGs should not be confused with

On the Banks of the Red Cedar

The marching bands for Michigan State University and the University of Michigan are both superb musical organizations, capable of stirring the passions of 100,000 fans on Saturday football afternoons, regardless of how well or poorly the team is doing at the moment. There is a difference between the two. Do you know what it is? That's right. (Good guess!) It comes down to their respective central pattern generators.

At the command, "Band, take the field!" the Michigan State band (figure 2.3) emerges from the tunnel at a frenzied rate of 250 steps per minute. (That's right—more than four steps per second.) Their CPGs are really humming. (It is not recommended that you try this at home, particularly if you're wearing a full band uniform and carrying a tuba.) Meanwhile, 70 miles down the road in Ann Arbor, the University of Michigan band marches in at a more laid-back pace of 208 steps per minute.

Why is this important? I guess it's because a close analysis might indicate that MSU trumpet players are likely to be about 5% leaner than their counterparts at the U of M. This will please their parents, who are footing the bill.

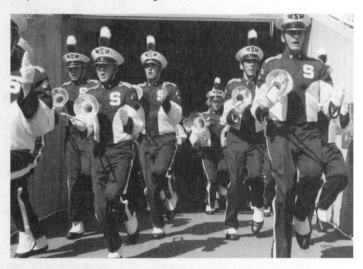

FIGURE 2.3. Central pattern generators, disguised as band members at Michigan State University, take the field.
Photo courtesy of Mark Hansen Photography, Ann Arbor, MI.

brain motor centers, which signal muscle contraction and control purposeful motor activity. Theirs is a different task. CPGs are assigned the specific role of subconsciously controlling the rhythmicity and tempo of that activity. They are distinct from motor control areas in the cerebral cortex that we can willfully command.

The volume and level of sophistication of research regarding CPGs has grown dramatically in the last decade. What follows is simply a quick overview of where this information has taken us. We'll start with findings in more simple animals and move up the evolutionary ladder to what is known about humans. Those wishing a more detailed examination of current investigations into the nature of CPGs can consult a number of in-depth reviews.[9] (Also, a warning: lovers of cats—and, for that matter, eels—may wish to skip the following sections.)

Lampreys

The lamprey is a repugnant, eel-like creature that makes its living by sucking the blood and body fluids out of other fishes. Perhaps to compensate for its lack of social deportment, this primitive vertebrate has provided researchers some intriguing insights into the evolutionary origins of CPGs.

The lamprey swims by producing waves of muscle activity, contracting sequentially from head to tail. Contraction of each of the segmental muscles is triggered by nerve cells located in the spinal cord. While each segment has to be coordinated with the next one down the line, there must be a time lag to create a wave. (If not, obviously, the entire set of muscles would contract simultaneously, rather than producing a wave. That would be like everyone in the football stadium trying to do the wave by standing up at the same time.) It turns out that the delay from segment to segment is about 1% of the total wave duration, and about 100 segments exist. Cycle duration depends on the swimming speed. If the lamprey is swimming at top speed, the cycle duration is about 100 milliseconds, meaning that the firing rate sequence of spinal motor neurons involves a lag of 1 millisecond between each segment and its downstream neighbor.

Control of this sequence of muscle contractions lies in the spinal cord itself. We know this because if you remove the lamprey's brain and then electrically stimulate the spinal cord, you still witness coordinated swimming motion. And, if you go so far as to chop the spinal cord into pieces containing only two or three muscle segments, electrical stimulation still causes swimlike activity in what muscle still remains. (You can try this in your spare time at home, best after your spouse has gone to bed.) On the other hand, the control of the rate of the entire system of locomotion resides higher up in the lower part of the brain stem (something called the rhombencephalic reticular nuclei). Artificial stimulation of these structures puts the whole tail into action.

This information in this most primitive of vertebrates serves as the foundation for studies of higher mammals. The lamprey is telling us that there are really two neurologic controllers of automatic locomotor activity that function in respect to time:

1. Coupled segmental oscillators in the spinal cord dictate a finely timed sequence of motor neuron firing to provide locomotion.

2. A central controller in the brain stem dictates the generation of tempo and force for the entire system.

Too, this controller must act in response to sensory input. (The lamprey has to locate and chase down its prey, for example.) And, needless to say, the lamprey out searching for unsuspecting fishes to suck dry gives no conscious thought to the matter.

So, this is the basic model of two-tiered CPGs, with an autonomous oscillator that fires at a constant frequency (that's the spinal cord CPG) and a calibration unit (in this case, brain stem centers) that adjusts this basic frequency in response to information from the environment. Now, let's see what we find when we move up the evolutionary tree.

Cats

Experiments performed almost 100 years ago indicate that a cat whose spinal cord has been transected still demonstrates alternating, rhythmic contractions in the muscles moving the ankle that mimic locomotor activity. They also found (remember my warning, cat lovers) that if you sever the cat's brain stem and then electrically stimulate certain centers below the cut, the cat demonstrates complete quadrupedal stepping. In some studies, animals are even capable of spontaneous walking. This confirms the dominant effect of spinal cord CPG in feline gait.

Alterations in speed of walking, trotting, or galloping can be produced by changing the strength of the stimulus descending from motor centers in the brain. This central modulator, located at the level of the brain stem, regulates the turnover velocity during locomotion through descending nerve fibers that influence the oscillator in the spinal cord. There seems to be little control from higher brain centers, however, since cats do not struggle with locomotion after these areas are damaged.

The basic model of the CPG (or CPGs), we see, is the same as in the lamprey. A rhythmic generator exists in the spinal cord that controls the stereotyped, oscillatory pattern of muscle activation for locomotion in respect to time. And a higher, more central regulator at the base of the brain sends signals down the spinal cord to initiate and dictate the power output of the CPG (and presumably the proper relationship of stride frequency and duration) to achieve a certain velocity of locomotion in response to sensory stimuli.

Monkeys and Other Nonhuman Primates

As one examines ascendancy of the evolutionary tree, animals progressively exhibit extensive development of higher brain structures, particularly the cerebral cortex. It might be expected, then, that higher controlling sites within the brain would begin to play a role as CPGs. Monkeys and other nonhuman primates provide some information on this point.

In monkey spinal cords, the evidence for an intrinsic CPG that controls the sequence and timing of muscle innervation for locomotion is much less clear than in the cat. The few studies of spinal transection that have been performed in monkeys have not shown convincing persistence of locomotor patterns. Some reports reveal no hind-limb stepping after the spinal cord has been cut. It has been suggested that as compared to cats, the influence of the primate brain dominates over spinal cord circuitry for locomotion. The purpose of this shift might be to free the movements of the upper extremities, since the hands and arms are more engaged in nonlocomotor activities than the legs are.

Human Beings

Not much is certain about CPGs in human beings. Their existence, location, and function have generally been inferred from studies in animals. What data are available come from investigations of those who have suffered traumatic injuries to the spinal cord or cervix or vascular strokes. Patients who experienced complete transection of the spinal cord very rarely showed rhythmic locomotor activity. This has led some to doubt the influence of a spinal-cord CPG in humans.

Sandy Stevens, who teaches at Tennessee State University, doesn't agree. She has had a good deal of experience dealing with rehabilitation of spinal cord injuries. Her take is that previous investigations did not provide the proper sensory input in their research models. "Typically, in these studies, a harnessing apparatus is used that supports the body through the use of a groin strap," she says. (One of her patients actually called this system a demasculinator.) "This certainly does not replicate the sensory experience of normal weight bearing during ambulation."

Her answer to this? Underwater treadmill walking.

> We find that patients with partial cord injury who have virtually no ambulatory ability can demonstrate normal walking patterns when supported

by the buoyancy of water. I can't help but conclude that this approach facilitates spinal cord CPGs in stimulating normal stepping patterns. The CPG is there. It just needs the right sensory stimulus.

Supporting that conclusion, electrical stimulation of the spinal cord in patients with complete spinal interruption at the thoracic level has been shown to elicit some stepping. Steplike activity is observed in human newborns, even in those rare babies with anencephaly (they lack higher brain centers). Rhythmic muscular activity is evident in human fetuses within 10 weeks of intrauterine life. From the studies in nonhuman primates, however, it is expected that higher brain centers might play a more dominant role in timing rhythmic muscle innervation during locomotion than they do in lower vertebrates. This evolutionary progression of the central nervous system has been described as a progressive *encephalization* of motor rhythms.

Humans thus appear to possess the basic CPG blueprint (see figure 2.4)—a spinal cord generator that creates the rhythm and sequence of muscular innervation to coordinate locomotion in clocklike fashion, and a brain stem locus that controls the tempo of the spinal cord generator. Both of these structures are magnificently intelligent. The former knows just the right firing sequence of motor neurons that will allow a 6-foot (2 m) human to run upright on two skinny legs without falling over. The latter has inherited the wisdom of ages past that select the proper stride rate and length that are optimal for any given running velocity. In humans, of course, we must consider the potential added influence from higher brain centers that provide cognitive input—that is, what we consciously command of our arms and legs. The difference between humans and lower animals lies in the limited autonomy of the isolated spinal cord to generate muscular activity. That is, as we ascend the evolutionary tree, the driving factor for

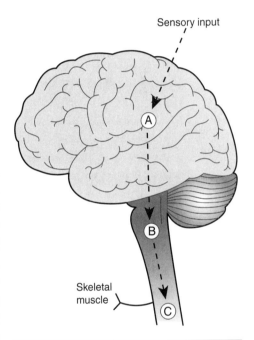

FIGURE 2.4. A schematic representation of system components of a human being's central pattern generator, based largely on information from lower mammals. The cerebral cortex *(A)* receives sensory information. By cognitive decision making or a subconscious governor, it influences medullary centers *(B)* to direct information regarding tempo and force of muscular contractions to the spinal cord oscillator *(C),* which coordinates the activation sequence of muscle fibers for locomotion.

Reprinted, by permission, from K. Haywood, 2008, *Life span motor development*, 5th ed. (Champaign, IL: Human Kinetics), 83.

the spinal CPG increasingly involves higher brain centers. Evidence suggests a decrease in the independent nature of spinal cord CPGs in human beings as compared to, say, the cat or the lamprey.

Internal Clocks

All of the neural structures and systems previously discussed operate within close time frames. Neurobiologists talk about internal clocks and specialized neural structures for timing that coordinate the automatic functions that let us run, bike, and swim. Whether such clocks are actually a part of CPGs or are separate neurological constructs is uncertain. Certainly, other structures within the human brain appear to participate in this CPG network that is so linked to the passage of time. The cerebellum, for example, appears to influence movement timing, since patients with disease in this structure have difficulty timing muscle activation during rapid limb movements. Patients with Parkinson's disease, who have abnormal function of basal ganglia, may tend to underestimate time intervals. This could be a sign that their internal timekeepers are slowing down. (Chapter 5 deals with the issue of time perception.)

It seems unlikely that a single master clock exists in the body, relaying temporal information to the different components of locomotor activity (the spine, brain stem, higher brain centers). After all (to cite an example that laypeople can understand), you can talk to a companion at the same rate while walking whether you are moving fast or slow. It's much more likely that numerous separate pacemakers exist within the nervous system that run at a similar rate. The intrinsic rates of such clocks could then be modified individually to adapt to local system demands. (A good pianist can play a 4/4 rhythm with one hand and a 3/4 rhythm with the other.) If you change the tempo of an action, the sequence of the action is not changed, but is simply condensed or expanded in time. This fits nicely with the idea that the spinal CPG of an animal is an intrinsic automatism, or clock, whose rate can be influenced by higher CNS structures, but whose basic firing pattern remains unchanged.

Entrainment of Locomotion and Breathing

One particularly intriguing observation that may have bearing on the organization of intrinsic clocks is that stride rhythm is often coupled with breathing during locomotion. That is, for a certain number of strides, there is a breath. This is called *entrainment* of ventilation and locomotion, and it has been observed in cats, dogs, horses, jackrabbits, gerbils, rhinoceroses, wallabies, turtles, guinea fowl, alligators—pretty much the whole ark.

Given this evidence for the evolutionary persistence of entrainment in the animal kingdom, it is no surprise that the phenomenon is also observed in humans who are running, walking, cycling, or rowing. In human studies, the reported frequency of the link between breathing and striding has varied widely. (In fact, some have found no evidence of entrainment at all.) Perhaps insightful, though, are the observations of Dennis Bramble and David Carrier at the University of Utah that the frequency of entrainment depends on the performance level of the runner. Experienced runners commonly coupled stride and breathing patterns very tightly. The most common ratio was a 2:1 ratio of strides and breaths, but at slow running speeds, this was frequently 4:1. However, in less talented runners, no synchronization of breathing and striding was observed at all.[10] (So, here's another laboratory exercise to try. Check yourself for breathing-striding entrainment during your next run and see which category you're in.)

The explanations for the link between breathing and striding during locomotion have generally involved mechanical issues. Gait, for instance, may physically constrain breathing, thus requiring the two to be synchronized. However, such mechanisms would seem to be less likely linked during the upright bipedal locomotion of human beings. Alternatively, a combination of effects of a single internal clock that links the two different forms of rhythmic activity is an intriguing possibility.

Does entrainment help performance? It depends, it seems, on which expert you talk to. Jack Daniels, who was introduced earlier in this chapter, thinks so. Given his extensive experience as an athlete (U.S. national titlist in the modern pentathlon), coach (University of Texas, SUNY at Cortland), and exercise physiologist (University of Wisconsin), he's somebody who should know. He notes that the best runners use a 2-2 rhythm, taking two steps (one with each foot) during inhalation and two steps during exhalation. If you're striding at Daniel's proffered rate (90 steps with each foot per minute), you'll then be taking around 45 breaths per minute. He believes this provides the most efficient ventilation of the lungs.

So, according to his renowned book *Daniels' Running Formula*, a 2-2 rhythm is preferred for the majority of a distance race. However, near the finish, you will probably want to breath faster, around 60 breaths per minute. Then you can switch to a 1-2 rhythm (take one step while breathing in and two while breathing out), or 2-1. Slower rhythms, such as 3-3 and 4-4, might be okay for easy training runs.

Daniels says to avoid a 1-1 pattern because the shallow breaths decrease actual lung air exchange.[11]

Jerry Dempsey is to respiratory exercise physiology as Jack Daniels is to distance running coaching. And Dr. Dempsey disagrees. "My argument, purely theoretical, is as follows. We have shown that the oxygen cost of breathing at maximal exercise in highly trained athletes can comprise as much as 15% of the total oxygen demand. This means a fair bit of blood flow is being required by respiratory muscles that is potentially stolen from locomotor muscles. So we need our breathing to be as mechanically efficient as possible. To me, the mechanisms in the brain stem are best designed to receive all of the input from the lung, chest wall, cerebellum, and hypothalamus in order to sculpt the optimal depth and rate of each breath to minimize the work of respiratory muscles. Higher centers, including the cortex, willing our breathing pattern to coordinate with limb movement would not provide the same level of optimization. So, in essence, I believe the brain stem of the runner is better equipped than the cerebral cortex of a coach to determine breathing pattern."

Distance runners Paul Norton and Jack Mahurin, whom you met in the previous chapter, line up with Professor Dempsey on this one. They both told me that anything that departs from just doing what comes naturally with your breathing is counterproductive. They think that concentrating on creating a certain pattern of breathing and striding wastes mental effort.

So, it comes right back to chapter 1's argument of the subconscious central governor versus our own conscious dictates, doesn't it? Should we let Mother Nature, with centuries of evolutionary practice, have her way? Or can we consciously adopt certain running (or in this case, running and breathing) strategies that will improve performance? I guess if people like Professors Dempsey and Daniels can't agree, we can safely call the answer inconclusive. But there may be a takeaway suggestion, too: Runners can try out active entrainment to see if it works.

Human Beings as Aerobic Endurance Animals

Before leaving this chapter, we should perhaps step back and consider a more basic question: Why have all these CPG systems and intrinsic clocks that help us run or bike or swim for distance developed in the first place? More to the point, why are humans, compared to our mammalian brethren, so good at aerobic endurance exercise?

Certainly other animals have extraordinary abilities to sustain physical effort. Like the white-rumped sandpiper, *Calidris fuscicollis*, who flies the 2,900 miles between the Arctic Circle and the northern shores of South America nonstop every year. Or the pronghorn antelope, which can sustain high speeds for 20 to 30 minutes, and whose ability to utilize oxygen at maximal exercise is almost four times that of the best human marathon runners. But these are isolated examples. In fact, out on the primate branch of the evolutionary tree, only human beings are capable of endurance running. Apes, chimpanzees, and monkeys can sprint, but only for very short distances.

How did this human ability to sustain exercise come about? What evolutionary forces have permitted 20,000 scantily clothed humans to cram themselves onto Route 135 in Hopkinton, awaiting the gun to signal their 26.2-mile run into downtown Boston each April?

Dennis Bramble and Daniel Lieberman are two people who have thought a lot about this. Writing in the journal *Nature*, they describe the anatomic and metabolic features that enable sustained exercise that evolved for *Homo sapiens*.[12] The list includes fossil evidence for musculoskeletal adaptations that improve energy economy derived from enhanced elastic recoil of the legs (long leg tendons, high longitudinal foot arches), factors allowing trunk stabilization (widened sacrum, enlarged gluteus maximus muscle), and optimized thermoregulation for hot African plains (effective sweat glands, lack of body hair, erect posture).

So much for the how. But what about the why? What selective advantage did long, slow distance running carry for our distant ancestors that now permits you to pin on that Boston marathon number? The fossil evidence cited previously suggests that our human ancestors first became equipped for distance running between 1.5 and 3.0 million years ago. Now, the hominid evolutionary branch diverged from that of other primates 5 to 8 million ago. The point is, then, that whatever Darwinian forces acted to make modern-day humans into distance running animals must have acted specifically on our closest ancestors (relatively speaking). When thinking about other aerobic endurance animals, this is evident, too. Clearly, distance running has developed independently in different evolutionary lines.

You might suppose that the survival benefit of being able to sustain exercise would come from an ability to scavenge or track down prey, particularly of animals who were faster—who could escape by sprinting away—but who could not maintain exercise for long periods of time. There are, in fact, primitive peoples today who chase down animals until their prey becomes exhausted. However, most contemporary hunter-gatherers rely on weapons—bows and arrows, spears—to kill animals they can't immediately outrun. These arms first appeared on the scene about 40,000 years ago, so we would have to surmise that selective pressures that favor distance running ability would have been applied before that time. But we really just don't know.

So, despite some good guesses, the full answers to our questions are not forthcoming. Our athletic endeavors today represent the heritage of millions of years of biological experimentation, of trial and error. We've inherited a magnificent clock-driven motor machine, one whose complex inner workings we can only faintly discern. Just where our capabilities for aerobic endurance exercise fit into this grand schema is not altogether clear, but you can bet that nature does things for a reason. And there may be broader forces and compromises to consider. I like the way Bernd Heinrich thought about this in his book *Why We Run*:

> A race is like a chase. Finishing a marathon, setting a record, making a scientific discovery, creating a great work of art—all, I believe, are substitute chases we submit to that require, and exhibit, the psychological tools of an aerobic endurance predator, both to do and to evaluate. When fifty thousand people line up to race a marathon, or two dozen high schoolers toe the line for a cross country race, they are enacting a symbolic communal hunt, to be first at the kill, or at least to take part in it.[12]

Notes

1. For additional information on the relationships between stride frequency and length in humans, see the following articles: Cavanagh, P.R., and R. Kram. 1989. "Stride frequency in distance running: Velocity, body dimensions, and added mass effects." *Medicine and Science in Sports and Exercise* 21: 467-479. Dillman, C.J. 1975. "Kinematic analysis of running." *Exercise and Sports Science Reviews* 3: 193-218. Grillner, S. et al. 1979. "The adaptation to speed in human locomotion." *Brain Research* 165: 177-182.

2. For those of you who were wondering, the human pattern of muscular activation and stride frequency or length with changes in velocity is similar to that observed in other mammals. This observation speaks to an evolutionary origin of our central motor oscillator (certainly not an unreasonable assumption given its subcortical, subconscious nature). However, differences do exist. In contrast to other mammals, for instance, primates (monkey, gorillas, chimpanzees, humans) have significantly longer stride lengths at a given velocity of locomotion. Animals such as cats and dogs, on the other hand, rely on increases in stride frequency to augment speed. Why should this be so? First of all, primates have unusually long limb bones compared to other mammals. Some have noted that primates generally possess a more arboreal lifestyle

(Except for you and me, they swing from limb to limb in trees). Maybe they are thus more adapted to leaping and consequently have a longer stride length for overground running. (Ponder this the next time you dash to the fridge for a cold one during a TV commercial.)

3. This is not, however, the entire story. Although minimal, variability in interval of striding time (stride frequency) during locomotion does exist. When these fluctuations between individual steps are plotted over time, we see what at first glance appears to be a total random variability. If you plug these into a computer that knows a lot about Fourier and fractal analyses, however, certain patterns begin to emerge. J.M. Hausdorff and his colleagues in Boston have done just that in a pair of studies that described step-to-step fluctuations as subjects performed sustained walking at a self-selected pace. Among the apparent random variability, their computers were able to identify temporal fractal patterns. That means that patterns of fluctuation in one time segment were similar to patterns in longer time durations. They found that variations in the stride interval could be statistically correlated to fluctuations in the stride interval several thousands of steps before. This self-similar rhythmicity in respect to time suggests that the variations in stride frequency during locomotion are not simply random events, but instead are under some form of biological control (from a central pattern generator). The biological meaning of such rhythms remains a mystery. What is their purpose? In this particular case, what evolutionary benefit would be gained by a certain regular pattern of changes in stride frequency during human locomotion? It is not clear if these regular fluctuations are a fundamental property of biological systems or if they represent alterations in response to environmental changes. We can't help feeling that some basic underlying principle that governs living matter looms here. If you figure it out, call me.

4. Serving as a backdrop to these considerations of firing rates of the central motor controller lie some intriguing notions of natural rhythms, or timing cycles, in humans. Indeed, what has been termed a *central resonant frequency of human movement* may actually be an expression of a more generalized, intrinsic biologic phenomenon. Velocity and stride rate during walking have been compared to the physics of pendulum movement. A pendulum requires external force to keep it swinging because of the dampening influences of factors like gravity and stiffness forces. In such physical oscillations, there exists a certain frequency at which such external forces are minimized. When subjects are allowed to self-select a walking pace, the stride frequency (1 cycle per second, or 1 Hz) has been found to be similar to that of a force-driven harmonic oscillator, such as a pendulum (0.92 Hz). These principles of physics may thus underlie rhythmic locomotor movements in humans, which could be indicative of the body's goal to minimize energy requirements.

5. Read more on dissociation by runners in this article: Morgan, W. 1978. "The mind of the marathoner." *Psychology Today* 11: 38-49.

6. This book provides a concise discussion of stroke rates during swimming competition: Maglischo, R.M. 2003. *Swimming fastest.* Champaign, IL: Human Kinetics.

7. Some good information on pedaling cadences during cycling can be found in the following articles: Marsh, A.P., and P.E. Martin.1993. "The association between cycling experience and most economical cadences." *Medicine and Science in Sports and Exercise* 25: 1269-1274. Padilla, S. et al. 1999. "Level

ground and uphill cycling ability in professional road cycling." *Medicine and Science in Sports and Exercise* 31: 878-885.

8. Gotshall, R.W. et al. 1996. "Cycling cadence alters exercise hemodynamics." *International Journal of Sports Medicine* 17:17-21.

9. Comprehensive discussions of central pattern generators can be found in the following articles: Dietz, V. 2003. "Spinal cord pattern generators for locomotion." *Clinical Neurophysiology* 114: 1379-1389. Ivory, R.B. 1996. "The representation of temporal information in perception and motor control." *Current Opinion in Neurobiology* 6:851-857. Marder, E., and R.L. Calabrese. 1996. "Principles of rhythmic motor pattern generation." *Physiology Reviews* 76: 687-717. Shik, M.L., and G.N. Orlovsky. 1976. "Neurophysiology of locomotor automatism." *Physiology Reviews* 56: 465-501. Zehr, E.P. 2005. "Neural control of rhythmic human movement: The common core hypothesis." *Exercise and Sports Science Reviews* 33: 54-60.

10. Bramble, D.M., and D.R. Carrier. 1983. "Running and breathing in mammals." *Science* 219: 251-256.

11. Daniels, J. 2005. *Daniels' running formula*. 2nd ed. Champaign, IL: Human Kinetics.

12. The evolution of endurance exercise skill in human beings and how it is related to that of other animals is treated in the following sources. The latter is particularly readable. Bramble, Dennis, and Daniel Lieberman. 2004. "Endurance running and evolution of *Homo*." *Nature* 432: 345-52. Heinrich, Bernd. 2001. *Why we run*. New York: Harper Collins.

TAKE-HOME MESSAGES

1. The central nervous system includes a system of subconscious central pattern generators with the following:

   a. An oscillator within the spinal cord that coordinates the rhythmic sequence of muscle innervation for locomotion.

   b. Higher brain motor centers that dictate the tempo of the oscillator and the force of muscle contraction that define stride frequency and length.

2. This system is under the control of intrinsic biological clocks that maintain a strictly timed sequence of muscle action and control pace of locomotion.

3. During running, the stride frequency and length selected by these systems for achieving a particular velocity is in some way most efficient, either metabolically or mechanically. Efforts by a runner to purposefully alter spontaneous SF-SL relationships may be counterproductive. The lesson here, as per the traditional coach's dictum, is "Pace, don't race."

4. In other sports, going with what intuitively feels best in respect to stroke or pedaling rates has not proven to be wise. Although coaches will argue, the best approach appears to be a process of individual experimentation to determine the best rate for velocity. Whether this corresponds to that which might be dictated by an intrinsic motor pacemaker remains to be seen.

CHAPTER 3

How fast can it go? The jet plane, the drag racer, the world's fastest man? Human beings are driven by a passionate quest to push the limits of performance. This is nowhere more evident than in our love for speed. Call us 0-to-60 people. This chapter addresses the role that intrinsic timekeepers play in making us run fast, pushing back the boundaries of sprinting performance.

DRAGSTERS, TIGER BEETLES, AND USAIN BOLT

Time and Speed

Let's think about physics for a moment. Power. You'll remember that power is taking a force (this happens when chemical energy is converted into mechanical energy) and moving something a particular distance in a given time. The force over a distance is called *work*, and *power* is the rate that the work gets done. If you lift a weight of 50 pounds (22 kg) up vertically 3 feet (1 m), you've done 150 foot-pounds (203 J) of work. If you accomplish this task in 5 seconds, the power output is 30 foot-pounds (41 J) per second. We express power in terms of watts, named after James Watt, the Scottish engineer who developed the first practical steam engine.[1] As he was trying to sell his new invention, prospective buyers wanted to know how many horses his engine would replace. He estimated that a draft horse could create a 150-pound (68 kg) force (like lifting coal from a mine) while walking at 2.5 miles (4 km) an hour. This calculates out as 550 foot-pounds (745 J) per second or 33,000 foot-pounds (44,740 J) per minute. This he arbitrarily defined, for all time, as 1 horsepower.

Today, machines have an amazing ability to convert the same amount of chemical energy into mechanical energy, creating movement and generating enormous amounts of horsepower in an extremely short period of time. The extreme example is the high-end drag racing car, which can blast through a quarter-mile race distance in less than four seconds at speeds over 300 miles per hour, or *mph* (480 kmph). It can generate enough power, 8,000 horsepower in fact, to reach a velocity of 100 mph (160 kmph) in just one second. In doing so, it pushes the driver back with a force five times that of gravity. To keep from achieving orbital velocity, the car has airfoils that push down on the wheels and keep them on the track.

How does it do all this? First, the fuel—that's the chemical energy—is not your 87-octane Sunoco regular, but a special brand of nitromethane that burns with an incredible kick (you probably don't want to light a match around it). The basic structure and function of the engine is the same as the Volvo's (pistons and all that), but in the dragster, everything is bigger. It has twice the displacement of the 1992 model. And all sorts of other modifications are present, all designed to instantaneously squeeze enormous amounts of power in just a few seconds' time. An air pump sucks oxygen in at a rapid rate to speed the burning of the fuel. There are also impressive sounding things like radical cam profiles, programmable ignition systems, and high compression ratios.

What about animals? This is a bit more difficult to address. To start with, how would a biologist studying this question convince an animal to run at top speed? And how could you be sure it was really running at top velocity? You would certainly argue, too, that the whole issue of maximal speed must be put into the context of how long the speed can be maintained. But having said all that, we know that certain mammals are speedsters, such as cheetahs and gazelles, who can approach running speeds of 70 mph (113 kmph). It's said that a cheetah can accelerate more rapidly than a Ferrari and can reach stride lengths up to 25 feet (8 m). Not quite like on the drag racing track, but still amazingly fast.

In proportion to size, however, lowly insects are the fastest animals on the planet. The speed title goes to the puritan tiger beetle, which can scoot after prey at a meter (that's equal to 80 body lengths) in a single second. These guys run so fast, in fact, that their eyes can't keep up, and they end up losing sight of their lunch. The cockroach is a close runner-up, generating speeds up to 50 body lengths per second, which is equivalent to a human sprinter reaching 200 mph (320 kmph) or finishing a 100-yard dash in less than a second.

The Human Machine

What about human athletes? They're machines, just like the drag racing car. When they exercise, they burn fuel with oxygen to convert chemical energy into muscular activity, creating power. Some aspect of power production is important for most sports. For the wrestler, it's the ability to drive a resisting opponent to the mat. For the road cyclist, it's a question of how long a certain level of power can be sustained over a particular distance. This chapter focuses on events that demand the all-out peak performance of that motor machinery. When putting their bodies into motion, what's the maximal power that humans can generate over time? The answer, as of August 17, 2009, is one which will drive an 86-kilogram man down a 100-meter track in 0:09.58. About 10 meters per second. That's what Jamaican sprinter Usain Bolt did to set the world record at the Berlin world championships, identifying him as the world's fastest man ever. (Afterward, I headed down to the high school track and, ignoring my wife's snickering, tried it for myself. My time, obviously impeded by a bit of headwind, was 0:26.28.)

How much horsepower did Usain achieve? Professor Vladimir Zatsiorsky, who is a biomechanist at Penn State, informs me that you can't tell. You aren't able to actually calculate horsepower production during sprinting since vectors of power production (directions of body movement) occur in multiple directions (vertical, horizontal, lateral), the contributions of elastic recoil can't be accurately quantified, and energy transfer occurs between individual body segments. Moreover, the magnitude of the leg muscles' power production in propelling the body toward the finish line depends on the portion of the race. Much more is required in the acceleration phase, although segment energy transfer and elastic recoil largely account for propulsion once a steady speed has been attained.

But how did Usain do this? What combination of physiological, biomechanical, and psychological factors makes his machine so incredibly unique? He and I use the same fuel (unless, of course, his future drug testing finds evidence of nitromethane). We both work with arms and legs. What special features give him the ability to generate that much power? How can his central pattern generator rev up with so much speed? This chapter explores the answers.

When Usain Bolt lined up at the start in Berlin, he had just one goal in mind—to maximize his power output for a very short time. He didn't care much about submaximal metabolic efficiency, glycogen stores, or oxygen delivery. Looking down the track from the starting blocks, he simply wanted to cover that 100 meters with the motor machinery going full blast.

In sprinting, then, the limits of muscular capacity to produce force might be expected to play a more pure role in defining performance than in distance events. That raises a whole new set of questions. Just how fast can the central pattern generator go? Since it never seems to actually come off the tracks, is there a brain governor involved here that dictates an upper limit of oscillator turnover during sprinting in the name of runner safety? How important is the tempo of stride frequency to sprinting performance versus muscular force production (stride length)? What happens if you cognitively change one or the other? What are the effects of training?

To start with, does body size have anything to do with it? If you're bigger, can you go faster? An interesting proposal was published in 1950 by the eminent English physiologist A.V. Hill, who concluded that any two animals that were proportionally similar in body shape would have the same top running speed, regardless of their weight. That is, a mouse should have a top running speed similar to that of a bear. The reasoning was that the mouse would have to take ten strides for every one of the bear's, but those strides would be ten times quicker than the larger animal's. Therefore, they'd cross the finish line together.

Well, that hypothetical reasoning might be based on sound mechanical ideas, but it doesn't seem to jibe with our common expectations. The biologist John Tyler Bonner didn't think so, either. He plotted the running speeds of animals ranging in size from bacterium to blue whales (this included results of a race created by a colleague between different types of mites) against body length. Not surprisingly, this approach showed that, in general, bigger animals are faster. Peak velocity of locomotion is directly related to animal size.

However, if you focus just on mammals, a somewhat different picture emerges. Look at the graph in figure 3.1, which plots the peak running velocity of these larger animals against the logarithm of body mass.[2] There's not much of a relationship to be seen. It would appear, then, that top running speed among mammals relates primarily to specific adaptations that equip them for high running velocity.

Note, too, that the human sprinter does not stack up very well against his fellow mammalian athletes. Although Usain Bolt can reach a top speed of about 30 mph (48 kmph) briefly during a 100-meter sprint, a pronghorn antelope can sustain 40 mph (65 kmph) for at

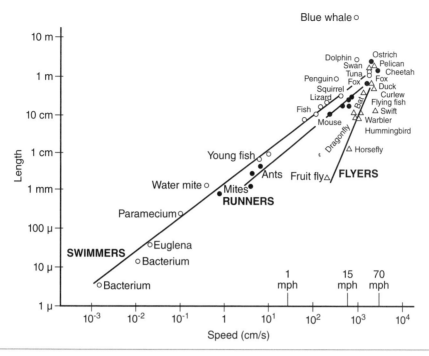

FIGURE 3.1. Speed of various animals plotted against their length on a log-log graph.

least 20 minutes. A greyhound can sprint 100 meters in 5.33 seconds, beating Usain's 9.58. The 200-meter sprint record for a thoroughbred race horse is 11.49 seconds. For a human being, it's 19.19. Indeed, all sorts of animals are faster than humans, even the household cat, who can achieve speeds of 30 mph.[3]

Empiric Observations on Sprinting

If you want to propel yourself as fast as possible down a 100-meter track, you can only do it in certain ways. For starters, there are two basic means—you can increase the frequency of your stride or you can push off harder to lengthen each stride. Your top speed would be governed, then, by how fast you can crank up the CPG and by how much force you can apply to joint extension (in this case, mainly at the hip and ankle).

Beyond this, however, things get more complicated. For example, you can achieve a greater stride frequency by either repositioning your legs more rapidly or by limiting the time that your foot is in contact with the ground. Besides applying force, stride distance can be lengthened with elastic recoil forces. The speed of forward propulsion—the direction you want to go—can be altered by applying different horizontal and vertical vectors of force. A number of extrinsic factors can potentially affect sprint performance, such as terrain, shoes, weather, motivation, and wind resistance.

Let's start this analysis of time as it affects sprinting performance by simply observing what happens to runners when they perform a short all-out sprint. Average sports fans who are sitting in front of the television watching a 100-meter sprint see a frantic blur of windmilling legs just after the crack of the starter's gun. Just when they have figured out who's leading, the runners burst across the finish line, and it's all over. If they play the race back in slow motion, however, this event of about 10 seconds can be broken down into distinct phases. First is the starting block phase, which is the time it takes to leave the blocks. The time of progressive increase in speed, or the acceleration phase, comes next. This takes up the first 30 to 40 meters of a 100-meter event. This is followed by a period of constant top speed and a late phase of deceleration just before the finish line is crossed. When Usain Bolt won the 100-meter Olympic gold medal in Beijing, for example, his split times broken down into 20-meter segments were typical of this pattern (figure 3.2).

As the sprinter's velocity changes during a 100-meter event, then, we can identify a time-velocity curve like this. Since the relative contributions of stride frequency and force production for stride length may differ for each phase, we can examine the running dynamics for each portion of the race.

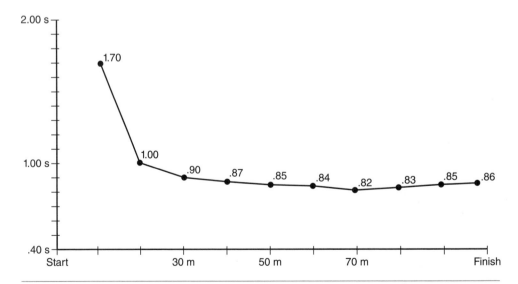

FIGURE 3.2. Split times for each 20-meter section of Usain Bolt's 100-meter sprint record during the 2008 Olympic Games.

Starting Block Phase

Obviously, the less time spent getting out of the starting blocks at the sound of the gun, the better. This should be particularly true in sprints of short duration, like the 100-meter, where hundredths of a second may separate the winner from the runner-up. Reports have indicated that sprinters' reaction times are not related to their finish times. And there have certainly been world-champion sprinters who did not start strongly. But in races this brief, it doesn't often pay to have a sluggish start. So, sprinters work hard to minimize their time getting out of the blocks.

When researchers study simple reaction times, like how long it takes to push a button in response to a light signal, the value is usually about 0.235 seconds. The time is greater if the responsive act is complex or if some decision making is involved. Simple reaction times in trained sprinters seem to be much shorter. A group of French investigators found that the average time to press a button in response to an auditory stimulus was nearly three times quicker for sprinters than for nonathletes (0.128 compared to 0.352 milliseconds, respectively), while physical education students had intermittent values.[4]

Interestingly, then, sprinters' reaction time (from the firing of the starter's gun to leg push-off) is generally very short. Reaction times at the start of a 100-meter sprint are shorter for elite runners than for those with less experience. When defined as the time between when the gun is fired and when 10 kilograms of force are applied to the blocks, 100-meter sprinters typically have about a reaction time of 0.15 seconds.

The issue bears importance, since track-and-field organizations have defined a start less than 0.1 seconds after the gun as a *false start*. They level out punishment—disqualification—based on this criterion. This assumes that any time lag less than 0.1 seconds is incompatible with sprinters' physiological reaction time. Therefore, their start would have preceded the gun.

Alexander Brown and colleagues at the University of Alberta analyzed starts for 100-meter events at both the 1996 and 2004 Olympic Games and found a relationship between reaction times and lane assignment. In these events, the starter fired the gun from a position inside the track and adjacent to lane 1. The signal and the voice commands of the starter were transmitted through loudspeakers that were placed behind each sprinter. This measure was to avoid any possible differential in start detection that might be caused by a delay of direct sound transmission. (That is, the sprinter in lane 1 would hear it first.) Brown and colleagues found that even with this system in place, the average reaction times of runners starting farther away from lane 1 were generally slower. The average reaction time in lane 1 was 0.160 seconds. For the other lanes, it ranged from 0.171 to 0.185 seconds. Out in lane 7, the mean reaction time was 0.185 seconds.

Investigators suggested that the sprinters starting closer to the starter had faster reaction times due to the greater volume and startle effect of the gun. (This doesn't seem out of the question, since the bang can reach an intensity of 180 decibels.) They pointed out that "the difference in mean reaction time for runners in lane 1 compared to all other lanes was not trivial, given the fact that first and second places in the men's 100-meter sprint final in 2004 were separated by only 10 milliseconds."[5]

Acceleration Phase

After the start, it may take the 100-meter sprinter as long as half the event just to get up to speed. It takes this long to overcome a number of forces that are acting to oppose the sprinter's forward motion, including joint friction, muscle viscosity, gravity, and air resistance. It's a very expensive start in terms of energy, too, since accelerating costs much more than maintaining a constant pace. Both the tempo of the CPG and the force directed per stride increase. That is, increases in both stride frequency and stride length contribute to the quickening of pace.

There is, of course, no way to get around this slower acceleration phase, although training may reduce its duration. The fixed contribution of time required to accelerate accounts for the interesting observation that a world-class sprinter can run a 200-meter event in less than twice the time it takes to finish a 100-meter race. For example, Bolt's Olympic record times in the 100-meter and 200-meter events were 0:09.69 and 0:19.30, respectively.

Constant Speed Phase

During the middle portion of the sprint, most runners reach and maintain a peak velocity. Studies of the athletes running at various speeds have been performed to determine the relative contributions of stride frequency and length to velocity during this portion of the race. At relatively slow speeds (below 7 meters per second, or m/s), both stride rate and stride length increase in a linear fashion with rise in velocity. Increases in stride length are, as expected, accompanied by parallel rise in production of muscle force. Above this speed, however, stride rate increases more for a given increase in velocity. To achieve high speeds (as much as 12 m/s), runners typically rely mainly on heightening the tempo of the CPG, increasing the rate of leg turnover. Top stride frequencies during this phase for highly talented sprinters are usually 4.1 to 4.7 steps per minute (or hertz, Hz) but can reach as high as 5 Hz (300 steps per minute), which is equivalent to 150 full strides. So, we can be immediately suspicious that factors that limit the top tempo of the CPG might be critical for maximizing sprinting performance.

The stride rate during sprinting competition is the same for both men and women. Here, we have at least some mechanistic insight: Sex-related factors (such as sex hormones) do not affect the top firing rate of the CPG. On the average, elite male sprinters have faster sprinting times than their female counterparts by about 7%. This has been attributed to their longer stride length and their ability to generate greater ground reaction forces.

Men's longer stride length is at least partially related to morphological differences, since the correlation between maximal stride length, body height, and leg length is generally high (with a correlation coefficient $r = 0.60$ to 0.70) among groups of both male and female sprinters. When measured in the laboratory with a 30-second, all-out Wingate cycling test, power is greater in males. This finding is explained by greater leg-muscle mass. That is, peak power adjusted for lean leg-muscle mass is equal in men and women. But, in one study, this couldn't be verified with sprinting. The investigators examined body composition and 30-meter sprinting times in 123 men and 32 women. (It should be noted that the subjects were drafted from college physical education classes. They were not trained sprinters.) Mean sprinting times were 4.4 ± 0.2 seconds and 5.0 ± 0.2 seconds for the males and females, respectively. Finish time for the 30-meter sprint adjusted for lean-muscle mass of the lower extremities was actually lower for the men than for the women.[6]

Suffice it to say that overall faster sprinting times for men than for women may not be explained simply by differences in body dimension or even composition (leg-muscle mass). Other factors, including elastic recoil (women are more flexible), fiber length, velocity of muscle contraction, and anatomy of muscle fibers (angle of attachment) may be involved as well.

It is probable that the power production during the constant velocity phase of a short sprint (50 or 100 meters) must be close to the peak power that one can generate in the laboratory on a 30-second all-out

Wingate cycling test, in which subjects are told to pedal as hard as they can. In such a test, power rapidly and progressively declines after about 5 seconds. It has generally been considered that the best sprinters can maintain a maximal effort for a similar period of about 5 to 6 seconds.

Deceleration Phase

Runners' speed slows near the end of a sprint, with loss of velocity from peak value of as much as 9% in a 100-meter event. The cause of this retardation has not been clearly defined. However, the toxic effect of accumulating lactic acid (a by-product of anaerobic metabolism) on skeletal muscle function has always been considered an important determinant. When velocity falls off while approaching the finish, a fall in stride frequency is usually responsible. Stride length may actually increase slightly. Coaches generally consider the most successful sprinters as those who slow down the least at the end, not those who start faster.

Performance determinants for the sprint can then be linked to each of these stages. Finish times can be influenced by reaction time (quicker times off the blocks), speed acquisition (shortening the acceleration phase), reaching and maintaining a maximal speed (the constant velocity portion), and minimizing loss of velocity when approaching the finish. Training strategies have been focused on each of these elements.

View from Lane 1: An Athlete's Perspective on Sprinting Races

Steven Headley came to Springfield College equipped with some Caribbean genes that help him run fast. Very fast. As in 6.24 seconds in the indoor 55-meter dash or 10.51 seconds for the 100 meters outdoors. Both results are good enough to make him two-time NCAA Division III national champion in 2008-2009. (He did, in fact, pick the right parents. In Barbados, his mother was a sprinter, his father a first-class cricketer.)

Steven and I sat in the campus library one day amid a crowd of bleary-eyed students cramming for finals, chatting quietly about what it takes to be a champion sprinter.

> **Headley:** When people watch a 100-meter race, they think everybody is just sprinting the whole time. But it's a lot more complicated than that. You can't run all out for more than about 4 or 5 seconds. That's less than half the race. The guy who wins

is usually the one who can sustain that top pace for the longest time, at the highest velocity.

After that, everybody slows down. At the finish line, it looks like some of the runners are putting on a burst of speed, surging past the others. But that's not it. What's really happening is those runners looking strong at the finish are actually not slowing down as much as the others. I really don't know what causes me to slow at the finish. Sometimes I'm not even aware of it.

So, you really don't want to accelerate up to top sprint speed too quickly at the beginning. If you do that, you won't be able to sustain your maximum speed as long, and you'll slow down sooner at the end. You don't want to be sprinting until 50 to 60 meters into a 100-meter race. Also, a fast takeoff from the blocks is good, but if you can't do that, it might not be a tragedy. One hundred meters is a long way. You can make up the time later. In shorter sprints (like the 55 meters indoors), of course, everything I've just said isn't quite so true. There's not much time to waste getting up to speed!

Rowland: Speaking of time, does it flow differently in your mind during, say, a 100-meter sprint?

Headley: It sure does. Ten seconds. That doesn't sound like a long time. But when I stand at the blocks and stare down at the finish, it looks like a long distance away. And it sure feels like it takes a long time to get there. Time seems to get extended. But that doesn't matter. I've got to be concentrating like mad the whole race. The mechanics have to be correct, the arms have to be pumping right, the body stable, the energy being sent down to my legs, keeping them low at the start. Just the tiniest mistake in all of this can cost you a good time, or even a win.

Of course, that kind of concentration is important in all sports, but with the sprints, it's a bit different. You have to be focusing just on what you're doing the whole time. You can't do anything about how your opponents are racing. It's not like football or tennis or almost every other sport in which you can try to outmaneuver or outsmart somebody else. In sprinting, it's just you.

Rowland: Does that mean that you don't think about the other sprinters as you head down the track?

Headley: Well, if you're up against somebody who just nipped you at the tape last year, you can't help being aware of him a little. But you'd never turn to look at him!

Determinants of Sprint Performance: Stride Length or Frequency?

So, what's more important to sprinters' performance? Is it how quickly they can move their legs (stride frequency)? How much force they can generate on leg push-off (stride length)? How can they best spend those 10 seconds that will get them to the finish lines faster? Training strategies hinge on the answers.

Not surprisingly, like most questions about the limits of physiological function, the answer is not altogether clear. Alas, the whole matter is once again much more complicated than we might have hoped. Consequently, researchers are lining up on the side of stride frequency, stride length, or both as being most critical to sprinting performance.

Just to start with, stride frequency and stride length can be reciprocal. That is, if you increase your rate of striding but do not provide a parallel rise in muscle contractile force to lengthen your stride, the length of each stride will shorten. And vice versa. If this occurs, increasing either stride frequency or stride length will not affect your overall running velocity. And if you're coaching your sprinters to work on improving one or the other, all their work will be for naught.

Then there is the fact that in providing an isolated increase in stride frequency (without an increase in stride length), the requirements for force production per step rises. That's because as stride rate increases, the duration of the support phase (when the foot is in contact with the ground) progressively shortens. Since the amount of force required to propel body mass stays constant, a greater rate of force over time is required for each step. So, it's not just the speed of leg turnover that increases as stride frequency rises, but also the rate of muscle force produced against the ground. Thus, as the rate of the CPG clock accelerates, the nervous system must transmit messages to the leg muscles to increase force as well, even if it is simply the stride frequency that is altered. It also follows that the runner is obliged to increase the strength of leg muscle contraction to effect both a rise in stride frequency and longer stride length.

In a particularly illuminating study, Joseph Hunter and his colleagues in New Zealand studied the mechanics of athletes who performed three maximal 25-meter sprints on a synthetic track that actually passed right through the middle of their laboratory. Sprinting velocities ranged from 7.44 to 8.80 meters per second. When analyzing the entire group of 36 subjects, a wide variety of ratios of stride frequency to stride length was found. The subjects with greater stride length had the highest velocities.

So, that means that stride length is more important than generating stride frequency when performing short sprints, right? Not so fast. When the authors examined stride frequency, stride length, and velocity within the three trials in each of the subjects, the results were different. In fact, the fastest trial times were related to the subjects' highest stride frequencies. The times bore no relationship to stride length. (This is consistent with research findings indicating that over the course of a competitive season, runners accomplish their best sprinting times with a higher stride frequency. Stride length doesn't change much.)

So, Hunter and coworkers found that the same runners used changes in stride frequency to effect changes in speed, while comparisons between runners indicated that alterations in stride frequency were more important. It seems difficult to reconcile these conflicting findings. The authors offered the possibility (which they admitted requires further examination) that "achievement of a greater sprint velocity via a longer step requires long-term development of strength and power, whereas step rate may be a more decisive factor in the short term."[7]

Based on these data, it is difficult to offer a firm recommendation regarding the relative merits of optimizing either stride length or stride frequency in sprinting training regimens. The data supporting a contributing role of muscle strength and rate of force production to sprinting performance, on the other hand, are quite convincing. As the preceding information shows, such factors may have a determining role in increasing both rate of leg turnover and length of stride during sprinting performance.

Cross-sectional research studies have verified the importance of a number of variables for muscle function. For example, significant correlations with sprinting performance have been reported for explosive strength (as indicated by height of vertical jump), strength on squat lifts, drop jumps, force production on a platform, and measures of both isometric and isokinetic strength. Findings in such studies need to take in account the muscle groups tested, since the contribution of specific muscles to forward propulsion varies in the different phases of the sprint.

A.I. Bissas and K. Havendeditis found that the ability to rapidly generate muscular force was closely related to 35-meter sprinting performance (correlation coefficient of $r = -0.73$). They found that the time required to reach 60% of a maximum voluntary contraction during strength testing in the laboratory accounted for 35% of the differences in sprinting times.

Important in this discussion, too, is a consideration of type of muscle fiber. Sprinters tend to possess a higher proportion of what are called fast-twitch, or Type II, fibers in their leg muscles than the rest of us do. These fibers are specialists in facilitating short bursts of high-intensity activities by their rapid contraction times and use of anaerobic metabolism. The calf (gastrocnemius) muscle of nonathletes is made up of about 50% fast-twitch fibers. The same muscle in a typical elite sprinter has about 75%. As expected, studies indicate a close relationship between sprinting performance and percentage of Type II fibers in the muscles of the lower extremities. Your proportion of such fibers can only be blamed on your parents, though, since muscle-fiber composition is genetically based and is probably fixed at birth.

If fiber type of skeletal muscles serves as a major determinant of how fast one can run 100 meters, we would expect sprinting performance to be largely inherited. Claude Bouchard and Bob Malina reviewed the research studies addressing this question and concluded that a considerable variability exists in the degree of genetic contribution to running performance in short dashes. This included reports of heritabilities (here, a value of 1.0 indicates a trait that is entirely genetic) of 0.83 for 20 meters, 0.62 and 0.81 for 30 meters, and 0.45, 0.72, 0.80, and 0.91 for 60 meters. You might conclude, though, that these values are pretty high and would therefore support the idea that muscle fiber type plays an important role in sprinting performance (and also that this portion of your sprinting skill is already fixed before you even show up for track tryouts).

The elasticity of muscles and their connecting tendons provides a spring effect that allows the sprinter to bounce faster down the track. The exact contribution of this elastic effect to running velocity is difficult to pin down, but it is considered to be substantial. Writing in the *Journal of Physiology* (217: 709-721), G. Cavanga and colleagues found that muscle contractile function of the legs increased in parallel with running velocity up to speeds of 5 meters per second. They suggested that elasticity of the legs was largely responsible for further increases in their subjects' speed up to a maximum of 9.4 meters per second.

Some interesting issues have been addressed regarding external influences on sprinting performance. For example, does the type of track surface affect sprinting times? If your high school decides to invest large sums of tax dollars in replacing the old cinder track with a synthetic rubberized surface, will the record you set for the 100-meter dash in 1970 fall? Maybe or maybe not. The issue is a complicated one. Synthetic rubberized tracks are more compliant—spongier—than the old dirt and cinder tracks. That might reduce the risk of injuries. However, if a track is too soft, it takes longer for your legs to rebound, and your sprinting times will be slower. On the other hand, if a track is hard, like concrete, there is no spring effect to propel you forward. Thus, a particular track compliance—not too hard, not too soft—will be just right for optimizing racing speed.

In 1977, Harvard University was in the process of building a 220-yard indoor running track with a wooden base and synthetic covering. They sent researchers Thomas McMahon and Peter Greene down to the gait analysis laboratory at Children's Hospital in Boston to come up with some mathematical models of running mechanics that would enable them to calculate the right degree of track compliance to be tuned to its runners. Their calculations turned out to be spot-on. In competition that year, the average best time of the Harvard runners was 2% greater than the year before. Other schools followed suit with similar improvements. Moreover, running injuries on the new tracks were said to be reduced by 50%. So, synthetic tracks may offer improved performance by augmenting energy rebound (and thus enhancing energy economy) and decreasing injury rate. (Of course, opponents would accrue the same advantages.)

However, the distance of the race might have an effect on these findings. Researchers at the German Sport University in Cologne found no significant differences in 60-yard sprinting times when the run was performed on hard, soft, or springy track surfaces. They concluded that the differences between track surfaces are sufficiently small as to have little impact on sprinting times.[8]

Steven Headley, though, has no doubt from his personal experience about the faster times he attains on newer high-tech synthetic tracks. "Improvements in sprint times can be due in part to better training," he says, "but there's no question that changes in track surfaces have a lot do with it. If I run 55 meters in 6.3 seconds at Boston University and then come home and do the same time at the Springfield track, people know that I really had a better day in Boston because the track there is slower."

What happens when you sprint around the curve of an oval track compared to running down a straightaway? Your velocity around the curve will fall off, with the extent of the decrease related to the sharpness of the curve. Researchers have found that in 200-meter competitions, runners are up to 0.4 seconds slower on a curve compared to a straight portion of the track. The amount of the delay is directly related to the curvature of the track. The greater the curvature, the slower the time. Thus, the runner in an outside lane has a potential advantage over competitors on the inside. One study compared sprinting velocities when subjects were running down a straight track with performances on circular tracks with radii of 1, 2, 3, 4, and 6 meters. Velocity progressively fell as the sharpness of the turn increased. It has traditionally been supposed that this occurs because on a curve, an application of a lateral ground-reaction force causes a decrease in peak vertical ground-reaction force, which is really the direction you want to go (figure 3.3). That is, if you have to turn, some of the force of your leg extension must be used for this purpose, which steals force away from forward propulsion.

Findings in this study, however, support another possibility. The authors found that you may slow as you round a curve because smaller peak forces are generated by the inside leg than by the outside one. This all has to do with complicated concepts of centripetal

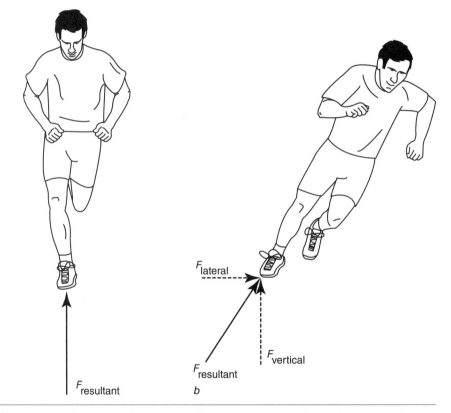

FIGURE 3.3. Sprinting around a curve increases lateral ground-reaction forces, stealing from those dedicated to forward propulsion. Shown here are force vectors for *(a)* running straight and *(b)* turning.

Adapted, by permission, from Y.H. Chang and R.J. Kram, 2007, "Limitations to maximum running speed on flat curves," *Experimental Biology* 210: 971-982. http://jeb.biologists.org/cgi/content/full/210/6/971

force, rotational velocities, and biomechanical restraints. Indoors, tracks can be designed with banked turns to reduce this effect, but this technique usually only works for a specific speed (for example, quarter-mile, or half-kilometer, competitions).

The authors noted that quadrupeds (four-legged animals) are able to decouple such constraints, and so they handle curves better. More than one researcher, it seems, has committed professional time to actually documenting that mice and dogs can round a curve at relatively greater speeds than sprinting humans.

What Limits Stride Frequency?

The starter's gun fires, and they're off the blocks! For the first 30 meters, the CPG system of each runner revs up, driving the frenzied running tempo at increasing rates. At that point, it plateaus off, and then remains pretty stable to the 100-meter finish line. There seems to be a ceiling above which the CPG pacer and corresponding stride frequency for a particular athlete cannot go. Why can't it go faster? What factor or factors limit leg turnover rate? Some of the observations outlined above would have us believe that one's ability to generate stride frequency might play a serious role defining sprinting abilities. If so, coaches and athletes might well benefit from an understanding of just what creates the apparent limits to stride frequency during these events. In trying to do so, we are clearly in terra incognita here—the descriptive or experimental research is extremely scant. But let's consider some ideas.

Harkening back to our CPG model from the previous chapter, we can consider components of this automatic oscillatory system, driven by internal clocks, that generates the rhythm, tempo, and force of muscular activity during the dash to the finish tape. Viewed in a simplistic way, the basic oscillator resides at the level of the spinal cord, the force and tempo are controlled from the lower brain centers, and, in humans, cognitive and subconscious cerebral input provides information as well. Where in this system might we identify factors that would define the upper limits of its cycling rate?

Firing Rate of the Neuron Pacemaker

You will remember that the principal actor in the CPG is the spontaneous, automatic, regular-like-clockwork electrical firing of single nerve cells within the central nervous system. The automaticity of these neurons occurs from movement of electrolytes (sodium, potassium, calcium) across the cell membrane. Although, like the sinus node pacemaker of the heart, these neurons possess an intrinsic firing rate, the rate of spontaneous firing (and therefore the rate of impulse generation) is clearly influenced by a number of external factors. In the portion of the CPG in the spinal cord, the rate of firing is dictated by higher brain centers (much as the sympathetic nervous system speeds up the spontaneously firing of the sinus node of the heart when you're frightened). What determines the maximal firing speed of these pacemaker neurons is not known, but obviously there must exist upper physical-chemical limits to rates of electrolyte movement across membranes (intrinsic control) and the commands of brain governors that influence pacemaker firing rate (extrinsic control).

Speed of Muscle Contraction

As noted previously, biopsy data indicate that sprinters possess a greater percentage of fast-twitch Type II fibers than distance runners (who have more Type I, or slow-twitch fibers) or nonathletes do. Type II fibers are particular adept at the kind of work required for sprinting performance. They possess a greater metabolic capacity for anaerobic metabolism, generate high muscular force over brief periods, and— pertinent to this discussion—they can contract at a velocity that is twice as fast as that of slow-twitch fibers. For example, the twitch contraction times for a cat's calf muscle are 75 and 40 milliseconds in slow- and fast-twitch fibers, respectively.

The greater the percentage of Type II fibers, the better the sprinting performance. It can readily be suggested that the upper limits of stride frequency could be defined by one's percentage of fast-twitch fibers in the critical leg muscles (the more fast contractors you've got, the faster your legs can cycle). In this case, the limiting factor for stride frequency during the constant speed phase of a sprint would be the number of fast-twitch fibers and the ability of individual Type II muscle fibers to speed up their contractions. The nature of that mechanism might be sought in an understanding of why Type II fibers can contract faster than Type I.

Nerve Conduction Velocity

That makes for a nice segue to a consideration of the possible role of limitations in nerve conduction velocity for defining maximal CPG tempo. The speed at which electrical impulses are transmitted in neurons is quicker in those supplying Type II muscle fibers than Type I. That's because the axons of Type II motor neurons are larger. (We know this from studies of neurons in the giant squid, whose enormous axons—up to 1,000 times thicker than yours and mine—provide it with lightning-quick impulses that generate explosive contraction of its mantle musculature for propulsion. Consider this the next time you're enjoying a pile of fried calamari.)

As expected, then, sprinters have greater velocities of nerve conduction than athletes in other sports. Can this be improved with training? Who knows? Studies have described increases, decreases, and no change in axon diameter of motor nerves following training.

Governor of the Central Nervous System

Chapter 1 discusses the concept that the brain, acting subconsciously, might limit distance-running effort to protect an athlete from the potential risks of overexertion (heat stroke, coronary insufficiency, muscle tetany). In this model, the central nervous system acts to create those intolerable sensations of fatigue that make you stop with your well-being in mind. Could this same self-appointed governor limit stride frequency and velocity during sprinting as well?

St. Clair Gibson and his colleagues thought this could be the case. While noting that no direct evidence for this exists, they felt that certain observations supporting the role of a CNS governor during maximal muscle contractions might apply to sprinting activity as well. This makes some sense, since we've seen that force production (both its extent and rapidity) also contribute to sprinting performance.

For example, if you contract your abductor pollucis longus (thumb) muscle as hard as you can, force output steadily declines over time. After 60 seconds, it will fall to about one-third of its original value. The same pattern is mimicked if you simply decrease an externally applied electrical stimulation to the same muscle by a third. This suggests that human motor units do the same thing. That is, they reduce their firing rates during sustained maximal muscular contractions. To St. Clair Gibson and his colleagues, this suggested that "the decrease in firing frequency may therefore be a centrally controlled mechanism to maintain force output while protecting fatiguing fibers from damage incurred by ongoing muscle contraction and ATP and phosphocreatine depletion."

They interpreted the progressive decline in power typically observed when a runner completes a series of sprints, one after the other, in the same way. The pattern of performance falloff in repeated sprints is, in fact, very similar to that observed in the model of force production over time in the single sustained maximal contraction of the thumb muscle described previously. Such decreases have traditionally been attributed to local metabolic changes, but St. Clair Gibson and colleagues contended that the decline in performance in repeated sprints is not necessarily tightly related to these factors. They proposed that the brain may sense that repeated sprinting with fatigued muscles might cause damage. In response, it may deregulate central command to limit force production and sprinting performance on subsequent repetitions.[9]

If such a governor did exist for stride frequency during sprinting, what adverse outcomes would it be protecting us from? That is, what possible harm would we risk by pushing stride frequency beyond some certain apparent upper limit? The most obvious possibility would seem to be risk of musculoskeletal damage. Increasing stride frequency shortens time of foot contact. Since total force must be approximately constant for each foot strike, the peak force the foot applies to the ground can be expected to be directly related to stride frequency (assuming a stable stride length and ignoring other factors, such as change in force vectors and elastic recoil).

If velocity is constant, increasing stride frequency does nothing more than shorten stride length (one is the reciprocal of the other). As sprint speeds increase, though, we've seen that both stride length and stride frequency can contribute. There may be some upper limit, however, in which the stride distance can no longer be lengthened, or even maintained. In that case, increasing frequency would be of no value to the runner, since velocity would not be increased.

Implications for the Sprinter

We can see that, for the most part, the essential factors contributing to top speed in the several seconds of sprinting time are reasonably well recognized. We know that the strength, explosiveness, and velocity of muscle contraction, flexibility (elastic recoil), and rate of leg turnover (stride frequency) are all important. It is recognized, too, that such factors may not contribute in the same way in the different phases of the sprint.

Particularly relevant are the findings of French researchers who looked at the contribution of leg strength and flexibility to velocity in each third of a 100-meter sprint in experienced runners. They showed that strength (as measured by half-squats with loaded barbells) was a predictor of total 100-meter time as well as performance in each of the three separate 30-meter phases. Explosive power, which was assessed by a countermovement jump, was also associated with both 100-meter time and with velocity in the first segment. A hopping test was connected to performance in the latter portion of the race. Those who had greatest leg stiffness increased their speed the most between the first and second phases, but slowed down more at the end.[10]

This study suggested that particular motor tests could be useful in identifying an individual sprinter's strengths and weaknesses in the different portions of the sprint. Moreover, its implications for specific training strategies might be effective in improving performance in particular race segments.

The bottom line, then, is that appropriate training regimens are best designed with the idea of maximizing all components of sprinting fitness. Traditionally, this is what coaches have done. Standard methods of resistance training (particularly weighted squats or dead lifts) have been used to improve muscle strength. They are designed to avoid increasing muscle bulk or decreasing flexibility. Speed drills (that is, those that mimic race conditions) are deemed essential. Plyometric exercises are commonly employed, although it remains controversial whether jumping on or off boxes is really useful in optimizing sprinting times. Skipping, hopping, and quick-recovery high-knee running are designed to improve contraction velocity, flexibility, and strength.

What about stride frequency? The preceding discussion suggests the importance of leg turnover rate in sprinting performance, but also makes the observation that a ceiling of stride frequency during sprinting seems to exist (perhaps beneficially dictated by a CNS governor). Can the intrinsic clocks that dictate cyclical rhythms of leg muscle contraction be convinced to go faster? Should they be convinced to do so? Is it wise? (We've already mentioned some potential risks.) How might one go about increasing stride frequency during sprints?

At the least, we can respond to the last question. A number of training methods have been suggested to augment stride frequency. The easiest is simply running downhill at a very slight decline. You can perform sprints with the wind at your back. Certain devices will tow a runner. Coaches have advised caution when attempting to increase cadence with training, however. They warn that musculoskeletal injury and damage from falling can occur, particularly if the runner lacks trunk stability or good form. As to whether these methods really work to increase stride frequency and whether any such increases translate into improved performance does not seem to have been well documented. (Some reports have confirmed training-induced increases in stride frequency, albeit with a compensatory decrease in stride length.)

Indeed, this last comment appears to apply to the entire question of whether sprinting performance can be trained. We are accustomed to the concept that repeated, activity-specific exercise (training) triggers adaptive physical and physiological responses that translate into improved sport performance. The magnitude of such training responses in sprinting, though, has always been difficult to pin down. Considering variability of individual performance and the fact that the differences between being super and mediocre are in the range of tenths or even hundredths of a second, it is difficult to document training responses, much less to identify the training methods that might be the most effective. Indeed, a strong genetic influence on being quick, as manifested by an abundance of fast-twitch fibers in a runner's leg muscles, leads many to suggest that a superior sprinting ability is largely handed down from the runner's parents. It is not simply a result of intensive and extended training.

However, the old idea that great sprinters are born, not made, has gone by the wayside. Most coaches would agree that appropriate training regimens are critical for developing sprinting success. Given this, it is surprising that very few studies have been performed to see if gains from training techniques that are designed to enhance muscular strength, explosive strength, and velocity of contraction serve to actually improve sprinting performance. A group of Belgian investigators did demonstrate that nine weeks of high-velocity training (with plyometric exercises, jumping, and hopping) resulted in improved initial acceleration, greater maximal velocity, and better 100-meter times, as compared to a control group. The only effect of training with resistance exercise was an improved acceleration phase. No decrease in overall sprinting time was observed compared to the controls. Other studies have had mixed findings.[11]

Is There a Speed Limit?

Through the years—and particularly when the Olympic Games roll around—scientists have raised the question of the limits of running speed. Just how fast can human beings go? Since recorded history, winning sprint times have continued to improve, but is there a limit? What's the very fastest that humans can propel themselves down a 100-meter straightaway? So, investigators plot world-record sprinting times against race competition dates, connect the dots, extrapolate to the future, and attempt to draw conclusions.

The issue is far from trivial. Indeed, it can be viewed from a variety of mathematical, physiological, sociological, and even philosophical perspectives. It has bearing on such weighty questions as sexual equality, ethics of genetic engineering, and the essence of what it means to be human. For this book considering time, it asks us to think about the maximal potential of a central pattern generator to drive a muscle motor against a few clicks of the clock.

Beating the Buzzer

Think about historical plaques for a moment. There's one at the University of Chicago where the old football stadium once stood indicating the site of Enrico Fermi's first achievement of a controlled nuclear chain reaction. There's one at 74 rue du Cardinal-Lemoine in Paris, where Ernest Hemingway wrote *A Moveable Feast* in his upper-floor flat. And one in Lexington, where the "shot heard around the world" set off the American Revolution. But for an homage to sports and time, nothing is more moving, more stirring, than the plaque standing in Armory Square in Syracuse, New York, commemorating—what else?—the invention of the basketball shot clock.

The inscription reads:

This clock honors the rule that changed basketball and saved the National Basketball Association. The 24-second shot clock, which put an end to stalling tactics that were threatening the league, was used for the first time in an NBA scrimmage organized by Danny Biasone on August 10, 1954 at Blodgett Vocational High School in Syracuse. In the first season with the clock, league scoring would rise by 13.6 points per game.

Reading on, you learn that coach Howard Hobson (Oregon State, Yale) first thought up the idea of the shot clock, but Emil Barboni and Leo Ferris were responsible for coming up with the 24 seconds. You had to get a shot off before it expired. It seems they took the number of seconds in a 48-minute game (2,880) and divided it by 120, the average number of shots taken in a game at that time. (In collegiate competition now, it's 35 seconds for men and 30 seconds for women.)

Basketball fans over the age of 50 or 60 remember what the game was like before all this happened. A team would get ahead in the second half, and the four-corner offense would begin, a contest of keep-away in which the leading team would try to stall the game out to the end. It included lots of fouling, and was incredibly b-o-r-i-n-g. You'd see scores like the 19-18 win by the Fort Wayne Pistons over the Minneapolis Lakers in November of 1950. Well, with the advent of the shot clock, the game picked up pace, and, so they say, the NBA was saved.

For sports history buffs seeking a pilgrimage, I understand the original shot clock is located at Le Moyne College in Syracuse.

What Do World Records Mean?

When Usain Bolt set his 100-meter records, he was dubbed the world's fastest human. No doubt, that's an electric statement—in the millions of years of human existence, no person has ever run that distance faster, and we were here to witness it. But what does this really mean in respect to the limits of what the human machine can do? What is it telling us about human potential? Let's consider two perspectives—two very different concepts that would, in fact, seem to be polar opposites.

Idea 1. A world record of running performance time is a numerical indicator, a quantification of the functional limits of the human body. The sliding of actin-myosin filaments in response to electro-chemical stimulation can only occur so fast. There is a maximum rate, based on biophysical principles, at which neurons can repetitively fire in the brain, at which electrolytes can move across cell membranes in response to electrical gradients to permit nerve conduction, at which chemical energy can be converted into mechanical work. Laws of physics, of chemistry, of biology place a limit on how fast the human machine can go. This is objective reality. World sprinting records are set by extraordinarily rare individuals who can take these processes to the extreme.

Idea 2. Every human athletic performance, including the world record in the 100-meter sprint, is a second-best effort. There is always a reserve. Usain Bolt could have gone faster. We know this because at the finish line, he suffered no critical body damage—his heart, lungs, muscles, bones, and brains were all intact. Our bodies (read *central governors*) protect us from the true risks that would occur with a maximal performance. It does this by diminishing signals from the brain that lessen the force of muscle contraction and by overwhelming us with disagreeable sensations of fatigue that cause us to slow down or stop.

Humans are machines with functional limitations, yes, but they are apparatus with a safety governor. World-record sprinting times are set by people with the capacity to make the most of these limitations.

Solomon-like wisdom from the Great Conciliator. Maybe both ideas are valid.

Forecasting From the Past

When people have plotted winning Olympic times for the 100-meter sprint against dates, they show what looks like a straight line of improvement throughout the years. That is, they report a linear relationship between year and gold-medal times. In the last century, this has amounted to a full second of improvement in 100-meter sprinting times for men. When these findings are compared between men and women, things get interesting. The slope of the line, or the rate of improvement, is greater for females than for males. In fact, Andrew Tatum and his research group in the United Kingdom predicted the two lines would intersect in the year 2156. After that, based on their projections, women would run the 100 meters faster than men. "Only time will tell," they conclude, "whether in the 66th Olympiad, the fastest human on the planet will be female."[12] (Whether this will actually occur, of course, no one knows. But, here's a clue. Based on a similar analysis of marathon performance by sex, it was once predicted that women would outrun men in the marathon by the year 1998.)

Alan Nevill and Greg Whyte, another pair of British investigators, claimed such analysis suffered from methodological pitfalls. With polite restraint, they pointed out that the linear modeling of trace performance cannot be correct, since it implied no ultimate limit of sprinting times. Moreover, it led to the obvious conclusion that sprinting performances would eventually result in negative world-record times. That would mean that the sprinter would finish the 100 meters a certain time before the starter's gun sounded.[12]

These authors suggested that, instead, performance records plotted as velocity versus date actually followed a flattened, S-shaped curve. By this analysis, they said, there are limits to sprint performance, represented as the asymptote of this curve. They thought, too, that the greater improvement in women's records reflected the fact that the more recent participation by females placed them on the accelerated portion of the curve.

Thinking about this, it seems obvious that there must be a limit, an absolute time below which no human will ever be able to run 100 meters. Here's the argument. Would you accept that a 100-meter record will never be less than, say, 4.0 seconds? Sure. Okay, how about 9.0 seconds? No, it's not unreasonable that someday that barrier will be broken. The conclusion, then, is that somewhere between 4 and 9 seconds is a certain absolute limit that will never, ever be broken.

Having settled that an ultimate limit for the 100 meters exists doesn't mean, though, that humans might not continue to improve 100-meter sprinting performance. If a runner has an accurate enough clock and the willingness to add decimal points, performance can continue to improve, even if an absolute lower limit exists. Let's just say that no man or woman will ever run a 100-meter sprint in 8.0 seconds. But, in successive Olympic competitions, gold medal times could be 8.01, then 8.009, then 8.0009, ad infinitum.

None other than Andy Warhol made note of this. In his *Philosophy*, the artist talks about his musing when watching Olympic meets. "If somebody runs at 2.2, does that mean that people will next be able to do it at 2.1 and 2.0 and 1.9 and so on until they can do it in 0.0? So, at what point will they not break a record? Will they have to change the time or change the record?"[13]

What is Responsible for Improvements in Sprinting Performance Records?

Some have suggested that increases in sprinting record times reflect improvements in the biophysical properties of runners (for example, improvements in the capacity to generate energy by anaerobic metabolism). This could occur from factors such as improved training techniques or early identification of talent. Societal factors could also be involved. Giuseppi Lippi and colleagues have written that "economic advances and broader coverage of sports by the media have contributed to enhance the base number of athletes, including those at higher levels. This has increased the chance that 'extreme outliers' will occur in a normal distribution of athletes, and may partly account for an improvement in records."[14]

The Italian physiologist Piero Mognoni has emphasized the importance of training in accounting for improvement of world running records. He points out some interesting comparisons of human sprinters with race horses, whose capabilities are more related to selective breeding than to intensive training regimens. Over a distance of a mile (1.6 km), a race horse can gallop 2.47 times faster than a man can run, but horse-racing records are seldom broken. Over the past 20 years, 1-mile speed records have increased by 11.2% for humans, but only by 2.8% for horses. The conclusion? "An inadequate improvement in training techniques seems the easiest explanation of the history of equine records."[15]

Other external influences have clearly contributed to trends of improvement in record-breaking sprinting performance. It has been considered that the switch from manual to electric timing reduced times in the 100-meter event by 0.24 seconds and in the 200 meters by 0.14 seconds. Also, before 1930, sprinting times were recorded to the nearest 0.2 seconds, to the nearest 0.1 seconds from 1930 to 1964, and to .01 seconds after that. Changes in nutritional strategies, track surfaces, and training opportunities have been influential. Sadly, we must also include on this list the use of illegal (as well as legal) performance enhancement substances.

What of the Future?

An undercurrent of sentiment in all such discussions holds that, according to Lippi and colleagues, "future limits to athletic performance will be determined less and less by the innate physiology of the athlete, and more and more by scientific and technological advances and by the still evolving judgment on where to draw the line between what is 'natural' and what is artificially enhanced."[14]

Also, on the horizon are the approaching dark clouds of genetic selection and manipulation that will tax our ideas of the meaning of sports talent and performance as they touch all other aspects of human existence. We're not there yet, but the number of genes identified as being associated with physical fitness and performance continues to grow each year. In 2008, Greek investigators reported that a piece of chromosomal material called the ACTN3 gene was more than twice as common in elite sprinters as in nonathletes. One could suspect that once this substance becomes covered by insurance, a million Usain Bolts could emerge.

Implications of the CPG Beyond the Track

Finally, we can use the example of Boston College football receiver Gerard Phelan to point out that firing the CPG up to warp speed is critical for sports other than sprinting. Phelan, football fans don't need to be reminded, was on the receiving end of Doug Flutie's miracle pass that beat Miami on that game's unbelievable final play in 1984. Trailing 45-41 with a mere 28 seconds left, Flutie directed the Eagles to the Miami 48-yard line. There, with just six ticks left on the clock, time remained for one last desperation pass. Flutie dropped straight back, then scrambled to the right. With one second remaining, from his own 37-yard line, he sailed a pass that seemed to fly forever, over the outstretched hands of the Miami defenders in the end zone and—plop!—right into Phelan's arms for the incredible touchdown and victory.

John Eric Goff is chair of the physics department at Lynchburg College, and he's clearly taken great delight in figuring out the physics that explain how this magical moment took place. If you're into heavy math, check out his analysis in *Gold Medal Physics. The Science of Sports* (Johns Hopkins Press, 2010). For the rest of us, here's the summary.

From the snap of the ball, it took Flutie five seconds to release his pass, and the ball was in flight for around three seconds. So, Phelan had eight seconds to put himself into position to catch the ball in the end zone, 50 yards away. Dr. Goff estimates that the acceleration phase of this sprint (remember, wearing 15 pounds, or 7 kilograms, of equipment) lasted two seconds, and this carried him 10 yards. With his CPG now at full blast, Phelan maintained a constant velocity to cover the remaining 40-yard sprint in less than six seconds. (A possible deceleration at the end is unknown.) Now, at this point, when you and I would have collapsed in exhaustive agony, Phelan had to look alive and gather in the game-winning pass.

Flutie's performance at the launching end, of course, was no less impressive. Just how did he heave a perfect spiral 62 yards to the exact right spot, into a headwind no less? Goff thinks that the angle of launch was about 38 degrees, with an ejection speed of at least 58 mph, enough to reach the end zone in three seconds. And, if the ball were not thrown in an aerodynamically perfect spiral, it would have encountered so much wind resistance that it never would have gotten there.

Some have considered this the greatest college football play of all time. We know, of course, that more accurately, it was just the synchronization of two highly efficient neuromuscular systems, their central pattern generators, and a pair of finely tuned intrinsic biological clocks.

Notes

1. He is not infrequently confused with Isaac Watts, the English clergyman who wrote the Christmas hymn "Joy to the World." His history has nothing to do with steam engines and is a different tale altogether.

2. Read about animal speed versus body size in the following sources: Bonner, J.T. 2006. *Why size matters*. Princeton, NJ: Princeton University Press. van Ingen, S., J.J. de Koning, and G. de Groot. 1994. "Optimization of sprinting performance in running, cycling, and speed skating." *Sports Medicine* 17: 259-275.

3. After Usain Bolt set sprinting track records in the summer of 2009, his performance was analyzed against members of the animal kingdom in the following article: Stracher, Cameron. 2009. "Usain Bolt versus the house cat." *The Wall Street Journal*, August 24.

4. Hamon, J.F., B. Seri B, and B. Camara. 1989. "Motor skill acquisition influences brain responsiveness in sprinters." *Activitas Nervosa Superior* 31:1-6. A study of city bus and taxi drivers in downtown Belgrade also suggested that quick reaction times can be learned from repeated experience (such as sprint training). These drivers, whose occupations require rapid responses to sensory signals, were found in laboratory testing to have heightened sensitivity to visual stimuli. (Remember this the next time you're trying to hail a taxi in a rainstorm in downtown Manhattan.)

5. A consideration of the effect of lane position on sprint reaction times can be found in this source: Brown, A.M. et al. 2008. "'Go' signal intensity influences the sprint start." *Medicine and Science in Sports and Exercise* 40: 1142-114.

6. Perez-Gomez, J., G.V. Rodriguez, I. Ara et al. 2008. "Role of muscle mass on sprint performance: Gender differences." *European Journal of Applied Physiology* 102: 685-694.

7. For further reading, see the following articles: Hoffman, K. 1971. "Stature, leg length, and stride frequency." *Track technology* 43: 1463-1469. Hunter, J.P., R.N. Marshall, and J.P McNair. 2004. "Interaction of step length and step rate during sprint running." *Medicine and Science in Sports and Exercise* 36: 261-271.

8. Read about track surfaces in the following articles: McMahon, T.A., and P.R. Greene. 1978. "Fast running tracks." *Science American* 239: 148-63. Stafilidis, S., and A. Arampatzis. 2007. "Track compliance does not affect sprinting performance." *Journal of Sports Sciences* 25: 1479-90.

9. St. Clair Gibson, A., M.I. Lambert, and T.D. Noakes. 2001. "Neural control of force output during maximal and submaximal exercise." *Sports Medicine* 31: 637-650.

10. Bret, C., A. Rahmani, A.B. Dufour et al. 2002. "Leg strength and stiffness as ability factors in 100-meter sprint running." *Journal of Sports Medicine and Physical Fitness* 42: 274-81.

11. References for effects of motor fitness on sprinting performance: Delecluse, C. 1997. "Influence of strength training on sprint running performance." *Sports Medicine* 24: 147-156. Dintman, G.B. 1964. "Effect of various training programs on running speeds." *Research Quarterly for Exercise and Sport* 35: 456-463. Wilson, G.J., R.U. Newton, A.J. Murphy et al. 1993. "The optimal training load for the development of dynamic performance." *Medicine and Science in Sports and Exercise* 25: 1279-1286.

12. See the following articles: Nevill, A.M., and G. Whyte G. 2005. "Are there limits to running world records?" *Medicine and Science in Sports and Exercise* 37: 1785-1788. Tatem, A.J., C.A. Guerra, P.M. Atkinson et al. 2004. "Momentous sprint at the 2156 Olympics?" *Nature* 431: 525. Whipp, B.J., and S.A. Ward. 1992. "Will women soon outrun men?" *Nature* 25: 355.

13. Warhol, Andy. 1975. *The philosophy of Andy Warhol. From A to B and back again*. Orlando, FL: Harcourt.

14. Lippi, G., G. Banfi, E.J. Favaloro et al. 2008. "Updates on improvement of human athletic performance: Focus on world records in athletics." *British Medical Bulletin* 87: 7-15.

15. Mognoni, P., C. Lafortuna, G. Russo et al. 1982. "An analysis of world records in three types of locomotion." *European Journal of Applied Physiology* 49: 287-299.

TAKE-HOME MESSAGES

1. Specific training for different segments of the sprint—start, acceleration, top velocity, deceleration—with attention to technical aspects of each is critical for sprinting success.

2. Sprinting performance calls for optimizing the velocity and force of muscular contraction, as well as cranking up the central pattern generator to full speed (maximizing stride frequency).

3. In the past, such capabilities were considered mainly genetically based, and it was generally thought that few improvements could be attained by sprinting training. Currently, coaches feel that specific techniques to improve each of these determinants, including increasing the peak tempo of the CPG, can enhance sprinting times. There is, however, little scientific documentation of these gains.

CHAPTER 4

It is one of the most intriguing—and poorly understood—phenomena in all the biological sciences. In their physiological functions, all living beings exhibit rhythmicity that is closely linked to chronological time. This periodicity is observed from single-cell organisms all the way up to giant mammals. This chapter examines how circadian rhythms influence motor function and, by extension, athletic performance.

NIGHT AND DAY

Circadian Rhythms and Sport Performance

1979. American diver Greg Louganis, in a portentous moment fore-shadowing Seoul nine years later, strikes his head on the springboard at the Olympic trials in Moscow. He blames jet lag for upsetting his coordination.

1992. Skater Tonya Harding attributes her disappointing fourth-place finish at the Olympic Games in Albertville to jet lag, another complaint on her list of saboteurs that have upset her performances, including traffic jams, the back of her dress coming unhooked, a loose skate blade, a broken shoelace, and an assassination threat.

2000. U.S. world and Olympic champion sprinter Maurice Greene, once the world's fastest man, explains that jet lag was to blame for his loss to Portugal's Francis Obikwelu in the 100 meters at the Gaz de France track meet. In 2002, he withdraws from the Grand Prix 100-meter event in France, citing jet lag as responsible for his mediocre time of 0:10.56 in the heats. In 2004, he again loses to Obikwelu in France, complaining that his body was very tired from his overseas flight.

That's just a bit of athletic folklore about jet lag. In the preceding examples, was jet lag really to blame? Or was it just a handy excuse? When traveling across multiple time zones to compete, international athletes can disturb their regular biological rhythms. This physiological offset might lead to disastrous impairment in their performance on the world athletic stage. (In this regard, they would share infamous episodes of vomiting, fainting, and questionable judgment induced by jet lag that have also embarrassed political leaders during international voyages.) But some experts don't think so. All athletes in international competition must understand and adjust for travel-induced interruptions of their biological rhythms. But how much does jet leg truly affect performance? No one knows for sure. This chapter is devoted to the question.

Circadian Rhythms

By now, we should be convinced that we humans abound in timekeepers. We've seen in the previous chapters that our internal clocks finely tune the sequence of muscular innervation that permits locomotion. They guide our pace in races of different distances and they help us parcel out the rate of effort during different phases of competition. Without our conscious effort, these smart biological timepieces adjust, for reasons not entirely clear, the tempo of oscillations of motor activity during exercise to some optimal rate. And, when called upon to deliver maximal effort, they can rev up the muscle motor to top speed. Even the pattern of variability in stride rate or length during running and walking appears to be under the control of some reliable timepiece. It's a good thing that the alarms in all these clocks don't go off every hour.

It turns out, though, that even bigger timekeepers must be considered. In fact, every living being possesses clocks that govern phasic increases and decreases in cell function that cycle with chronological time. Since such patterns usually approximate a day's duration, they are termed *circadian rhythms*, from the Latin *circa* (about) and *dies* (day). They're evident throughout both the plant and animal kingdoms, indicating that these rhythms are a central feature of living matter. However, why our tissues do their work with an eye on the clock (unlike you or me, of course) remains an unsolved mystery.

The clocks that dictate circadian rhythms have no particular regard for athletic competition. But they do govern phasic changes in physiological functions that have important bearing on motor performance. Muscle strength, thermoregulatory mechanisms, cardiac output, even motivation all naturally and predictably change throughout the course of a day. So, the time of day when athletes train or compete may be critically important. We should expect that particular times of the day (or night) will optimize performance outcomes. Recognizing the characteristics of circadian rhythms as they relate to motor performance, then, just might prove beneficial to the competing athlete.

This chapter first briefly reviews what we know about circadian rhythms, their nature and mechanism. It then considers how these rhythms influence both physiological variables and specific outcomes of motor performance. Finally, it explores what happens to athletic performance when circadian rhythms are disturbed, such as the problem of jet lag when athletes travel great distances to compete.

History of the Circadian Rhythm

Paris, the summer of 1814, about 8:00 in the evening. Julien-Joseph Virey has just finished his duties as head pharmacist at the Val-de-Grâce hospital, and he is now roaming the hospital wards. "How many have died today?" he asks the clerk. "What time did they pass away?" He carefully records the answers in his notebook.

Professor Virey was working on his doctoral thesis, which he eventually titled "Ephemerides of the Human Life or Research on the Daily Revolution and the Periodicity of Its Phenomena in Health and Diseases." In this work, he presented a catalogue of known observations of 24-hour rhythms in both plants and animals and added his own observations of the daily patterns of patient deaths. He found these to demonstrate regular peaks of incidence at 6:00 a.m. and 10:00 p.m. This pattern has been replicated by contemporary studies as well.

Such regular biological oscillations had been observed by many before Virey's time, but his thesis was so significant (and unpopular with his peers) because of his claim that these rhythms were intrinsic to the organism, rather than simply a response to external stimuli. Since he turned out to be correct, it has been suggested that he should be credited as the true founder of the field of chronobiology, the science of biological rhythms.[1] This distinction came too late, however, since he died in Paris in 1846, unappreciated by his colleagues.

(Professor Virey was, in fact, not very popular with his peers, even when alive. Though obviously highly intelligent—he was also a naturalist, anthropologist, author, and philosopher—he never gained much favor with the scientific community. That was reportedly due mainly to his "naïve and wordy writing," indecisiveness, poor reasoning skills, and unpopular ideas. Indeed, one of the reviewers of his thesis commented, "This is the way, Mr. Virey, that one delivers medicine to public mockery and to the scorn of scholars."[1])

What was Virey talking about? Suppose you recognize that body temperature varies periodically and predictably over the course of a day, increasing during the day and falling at night. You might conclude, not unreasonably, that this rhythmic oscillation is simply a response of the brain's thermoregulatory centers to sleeping, fatigue, or maybe ambient temperature. But Virey contended that an endogenous rhythm to body temperature exists that is located within the organism, independent of outside forces. His opponents countered that these changes are simply due to the influences of external stimuli.

This debate went on for a good many years, and it wasn't until more than 100 years later that another Frenchman, a 23-year-old geologist named Michel Siffre, finally provided proof of the intrinsic nature of biological rhythms. Siffre figured that the best way to find the answer was to see what happened to body rhythms when a human was totally isolated from environmental influences, or even from the knowledge of what time it was. So, in 1962, he descended 375 feet (115 m) beneath the ground to spend two months by himself, camped out in a tent on an underground glacier in the Scarasson cavern in northern Italy. There in the darkness and cold, he was fully unaware of time, totally isolated from humanity except for a daily telephone call to supporters at the surface. His goal, besides geological research, was to see if his perceptual notion of time, governed by his physical needs for sleeping and eating, would be altered or dissociated from actual clock time. "My aim," he said, "was mainly to accomplish a kind of subterranean 'hibernation' that would fulfill a new research in human psycho-bio-physiology." (A lofty goal to be sure. Detractors claimed it was nothing but a self-engrandizement stunt.)[2]

For 60 days, he suffered bitter cold, dripping humidity, dark, loneliness, and terrifying rock slides, without any knowledge of time, day, or night. His diary records increasing bouts of depression, memory loss, visual hallucinations, dizzy spells, and severe back pain. (One entry about seeing pictures of his old girlfriends shows he was getting a bit nutty: "Farewell, dear girls. Farewell, the memories of my sentimental life. How I would like to hear your voices. Time no longer means anything to me.")

After he was dragged semiconscious to the surface when his ordeal ended, his estimation of duration for events in the cavern had become wildly distorted. But what had not changed, and in fact had remained quite steady, was his *nycthemeral rhythm*, the periodic duration of combined waking and sleeping periods within 24 hours. That is, even though one sleeping period might be much shorter than another, he compensated by making changes in the time he was awake. The overall combination of time spent awake and asleep did not change. Not only that, but the duration of this nycthemeral rhythm was a bit longer than a day at 24 hours and 31 minutes. With no clues whatsoever of clock time as measured by the rotation of the earth or light-dark cycles of day and night, his body had kept to a strict timetable. However, his was slightly longer than the solar day. Here was evidence in humans, previously indicated in plants and animals, of the intrinsic nature of circadian rhythms.

Later on, too, it was hard to argue against those who were clever enough to demonstrate the actual site of the pacemaker in animals that drove biological rhythms (the suprachiasmatic nucleus of the brain, for example) and to later identify particular genes that directed the running of the clock. Such rhythms were clearly generated by innate biological timekeepers.

With this point settled, the field of chronobiology took off. Aspects of biological rhythms have since become important to fields as diverse as medical practice, molecular genetics, ecology, engineering, and neuroscience. Indeed, another scientific field that encompasses as many different disciplines under its umbrella probably doesn't exist. No fewer than 14 international societies are devoted to the study, and workers in this field can consult several journals that exclusively publish articles about biological rhythms. According to a Medline search, 20,603 articles were published with the key words *circadian rhythms* between 1996 and 2008. The field is immense, filled with both intriguing scientific mystery and promise. The following section touches just a small portion of it.

Nature of Biological Rhythms

Rhythmicity—a regular, predictable, phasic variation over time—has been observed in the functions of virtually every living being in which it has been investigated. Single-celled organisms, like the *gonyaulax*, demonstrate rhythmic bioluminescence as they glow on the ocean's surface. Crickets chirp in diurnal rhythms to attract a mate. Bears are programmed to hibernate in cyclical periods with the seasons.

Most biological rhythms in humans are diurnal (that is, their cycles vary over a day's time). If you are like most people, a toothache is least painful right after lunch, your zeal to reproduce peaks at 10:00 p.m.,

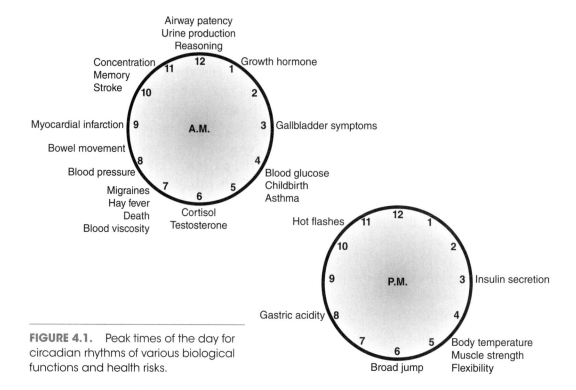

FIGURE 4.1. Peak times of the day for circadian rhythms of various biological functions and health risks.

your bladder fills more slowly when you're asleep (thank goodness), and you solve problems best at noon. Because of phasic changes in the water content of your intervertebral disks, you are tallest at 7:30 in the morning. And when the moon is closest to a position overhead, you weigh less, due to shifting gravitational effects (figure 4.1).[3]

All biological rhythms demonstrate two defining characteristics:

1. In a constant environment, as was observed during Siffre's adventure, biological functions vary with an intrinsic periodicity. Most approximate 24 hours (circadian), but others can vary in respect to the tides (circatidal), the month (circalunar), the year (circannual). They may even be longer, such as the 13-year reproductive cycle of the cicada. This endogenous, phasic change in function is termed the *free-running period*. As we discuss later on, these intrinsic rhythms are considered to be genetically controlled. They tend to be quite precise, some varying less than a few tenths of a percent in duration.

2. The intrinsic periodicity can be changed, or entrained, to fit that relating to extrinsic, or environmental, cues. Most commonly, this is the light-dark cycle in the course of a day (photic entrainment). In the natural world, the circadian rhythm of most functions thereby shifts to a more precise 24-hour clock

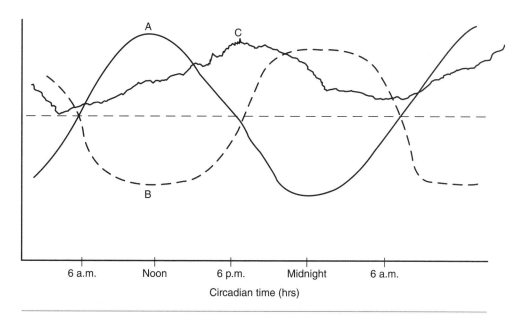

FIGURE 4.2. Examples of biological rhythms entrained to a ratio of light and dark during a solar cycle (24 hours). Line A shows the solar cycle, with the height of the sun above the horizon (horizontal dashed line), line B shows locomotor activity of a nocturnal hamster, and line C shows core body temperature.

(figure 4.2). Some interesting nonphotic entraining agents also exist, including cyclical changes in temperature (particularly in plants), song (birds), availability of food, and even social triggers in some animals.

So, in a dark cave, isolated from the normal light cycle of night and day, body temperature waxes and wanes following the directives of an internal clock that is set to about 24 hours and 15 minutes. If you leave the cave, however, your clock gets reset to a 24-hour periodicity that is linked to light changes in a chronological, astronomical day.

It is important to note, then, that although they have an intrinsic clock, biological rhythms operate in the real world by adapting to times defined by extrinsic stimuli. The central importance of biological timekeepers lies in their ability to adapt functions of the organism to geophysical cycles in their environment, not simply to generate their own intrinsic rhythm. It would seem, then, that both sides of historic debate regarding the nature of biological rhythms were correct: Regular phasic change in biological function is an intrinsic property of all living matter, but these rhythms are altered by extrinsic sensory input. The reason for this dualistic control is obscure. In this regard, it is intriguing (indeed, very puzzling) to note that in the temporal organization of biological rhythms, regardless of cycle duration or organism, the timing of the endogenous pacemaker is almost (but not quite) the same as that to which it entrains in response to environmental cues.[4]

Setting the Biological Clock

Where are these biological clocks? And who sets them? As noted before, it was only when these questions began to be answered by some clever investigators that convincing evidence emerged for the inherent nature of biological rhythms.

If you destroy the suprachiasmatic nucleus (SCN) in the brain of a rat, its circadian rhythms of drinking, physical activity, and certain hormonal functions are eliminated. And if you transplant the SCN of rat A into rat B (another fun home project), the latter develops the biological rhythms of the former. If you take out an animal's SCN (it's about the size of a BB) and put it in a test tube, it still continues to fire clocklike impulses. Additional studies have confirmed the SCN as the master biological pacemaker in mammals (and presumably in humans); other tissues may have subsidiary timekeepers, however. Some investigations have suggested that a great many individual cells (perhaps all of them) in mammals possess timekeeping abilities, but these are subservient to the SCN.[4]

These biological clocks must act to control gene expression and activity of transcribed proteins. In fact, a number of these clock-controlled genes have been identified. It is notable—and probably meaningful, in some mysterious way—that the subjects selected for such studies are common household nuisances (fruit flies, molds, and mice).

Importance of Biological Rhythms

The roots of rhythmic biological behavior that are linked to geophysical events (particularly the passage of the sun in a day's time) lie in humanity's distant past. They remain as part of our genetic heritage. From a Darwinian perspective, then, such rhythms must be interpreted as proffering certain survival advantages during the course of evolutionary progression. But what are they?

In many examples of biological rhythms, this is obvious. Reduction of metabolic demands coincide with a period of decreased food availability (hibernation). Intrinsic clocks adjust feeding times when food is accessible (honeybees). The same timekeepers are used for celestial navigation during bird migration. Serum glucocorticoid levels increase during times of high physical activity (rodents). The function of internal rhythms in response to geophysical events allows animals to anticipate, rather than simply respond to, these critical periods.

Other rhythms are harder to explain. Why should joint flexibility be greatest between 4:00 and 6:00 in the afternoon? Why does the stickiness of blood platelets peak just when you're getting up in the morning? Why can most people concentrate better between 10:00 a.m. and noon? Perhaps some clocks represent only vestigial remnants of functions that once upon a time bore importance.

The meaning of free-running biological rhythms remains a mystery, too. After all, we do not live in caves. And why do intrinsic rhythms (almost) match the entrained rhythm of chronological time (where the advantages of biological rhythms seem to be most evident)? Much has been learned about biological rhythms, but many mysteries remain.

Although biological rhythms are presumably expressions of adaptive mechanisms from our dim evolutionary past, their effect on behavior and physiology clearly has bearing for present human welfare. These diurnal variations help us consider the safety and performance of military personnel, shift workers, long-distance truck drivers, resident physicians, and astronauts in space. It has been contended that circadian rhythms (or particularly their interruption) have contributed to human disasters (which characteristically occur at night), such as the nuclear accidents at Chernobyl and Three Mile Island, the Exxon Valdez oil spill, and traffic fatalities. Human illness also exhibits circadian rhythmicity. Strokes and heart attacks occur most frequently between 6:00 a.m. and noon, asthma symptoms are worse in the evening, and certain drug treatments are more efficacious at particular times of day.

Circadian Rhythms and the Athlete

Count up the number of physiological functions that go into any particular athletic performance. Like a 10K road race, for instance. All the biochemical events that make up muscular contraction, the factors contributing to the coordination of muscular activity, the neurological innervation, the thermoregulatory mechanisms, the circulatory response, lung function, blood volume, cognitive and central command, motivation. By now, you're beginning to lose count! Next, consider that each of these many factors is attached to an intrinsic clock that causes function to vary periodically in a regular, sine-wave fashion over a 24-hour period. They increase and decrease in a constant periodicity, but each function does not necessarily reach a peak at the same time during a solar day. The conclusion? Circadian rhythms can be expected to weigh heavily on athletic performance and maybe even respond to training. Is this, in fact, true? And, if so, how can athletes time their training regimens and schedule competitions to best take advantage of peak periods of function that determine physical capacity? The following section considers the answers to these questions.

Athletes, who are always looking for a competitive edge, have had no small interest in the potential relevance of intrinsic circadian rhythms for sports performance. The result has been a considerable volume of research over the years that has examined the biological periodicity of both physiological variables and performance outcomes. In 1997, Thomas Reilly and his colleagues at John Moores University at Liverpool published a marvelous book titled *Biological Rhythms and Exercise* (Oxford University Press) that reviewed the published information on this subject. Updates have been forthcoming from this group since.[5] These publications, which are highly recommended, are available to readers who wish a detailed assessment of the research literature. I will endeavor to summarize what we know about biological rhythms and sports performance, supplementing those reviews with data from studies that are even more recent.

As we survey this information, it will be apparent that diurnal patterns of physiological and performance markers do appear to exist. But some important questions need to be considered:

- Do temporal peaks in function and performance truly reflect endogenous biological clocks, or are they simply responses to extrinsic environmental factors?

- If they are intrinsic in origin, are these biological changes of sufficient magnitude to bear importance to athletes compared to the influences of controlled factors, such as training regimens, equipment, and diet?

- How much individual variability exists in performance-related biological rhythms? Can findings in group data necessarily be applied to specific athletes?

It will become immediately evident upon perusing these data that the answers to such questions are not entirely at hand. Obviously, though, if recognizing phasic changes in physiological function and sports performance is useful for athletes, these insights are needed.

Physiological and Metabolic Variables

Virtually every form of physiological function demonstrates temporal rhythmicity. Most forms are circadian in nature, rising and falling in a sine wave throughout the course of the solar day. Such rhythms can thus be characterized not only by their duration but also by the amplitude of these phasic swings (how much the factor changes over the course of a day), as well as by the times of greatest and lowest activity during a 24-hour period.

Most of the physiological factors that contribute to physical performance demonstrate a peak activity in the late afternoon and early evening. It has been suspected that such patterns are driven by their link to phasic changes in core body temperature. Psychological variables that are expected to influence sports performance, on the other hand, tend to peak earlier in the day. In considering the timing of peak activity of such variables, then, one is confronted with the extraordinary complexity of the critical determinants of athletic performance.

Core Body Temperature

Core body temperature is normally regulated within narrow limits by hypothalamic centers in the brain that control gain and loss of body heat. During the course of 24 hours of normal life activities, however, measurements by rectal thermometer or gastrointestinal pill telemetry indicate a regular diurnal change in this temperature. If you are like most people, you are warmest around 6:00 p.m., with a temperature of around 37.2 degrees C. Levels then decline until you are coolest (about 36.3 degrees C) early in the morning while you're still asleep (4:00 a.m.).

This rhythmic change in core temperature reflects the combined effects of at least three factors: one internal variable (an endogenous biological rhythm driven by the SCN) and the combined influences of two extrinsic variables (the cycle of sleeping and waking and elevations in metabolic processes as you perform physical and mental tasks). To determine the relative influence of the intrinsic biological clock itself, you can experimentally place subjects in a constant routine, preventing them from sleeping and keeping them quiet and sedentary. When you do this, the daily rhythm of core temperature is unchanged, but the amplitude of 24-hour variation is somewhat reduced.

This information has led investigators to consider the circadian rhythm of core temperature one of the best examples of endogenous biological rhythms and, more specifically, an indirect indicator of

SCN activity (the latter being particularly difficult to study in intact humans!). Some have suggested, too, that circadian rhythms of core temperature may be the driving force behind other physiological rhythms that peak at the same time of day, since body temperature has a direct influence on a number of these. Moreover, in a number of cases, such a link might be expected to improve motor performance. Velocity of nerve conduction, for example, increases by 2.4 meters per second for each rise in body temperature of 1 degree C. Enzymatic activity in metabolic processes is accelerated as temperature increases. Elevations in body temperature may positively influence flexibility and contractile function of muscles and tendons.

On the other hand, we know that a rise in total body temperature, particularly when combined with high ambient-heat conditions, not only impairs performance in sustained exercise, but also poses a risk for heat injury (heat exhaustion, heat stroke). Accumulation of body heat is an anathema to the distance athlete. Anything that would add to body heat, be it a hot July afternoon or a circadian peak in core temperature, would be disadvantageous to a 10K finish time.

Thinking ahead to the next section on performance, then, you might predict that, based on a higher muscle temperature, you'd do best in short-burst activities like sprinting during the early evening. But if periodicity in sustained forms of exercise depends on the rhythm of core temperature, the opposite should be seen in aerobic endurance sports. Daily periodicity of performance in the heat in distance events (running and cycling), which is negatively affected by rises in core temperature, might be predicted to be opposite to that of circadian rhythm of core temperature. Best performances would be in the morning.

It's obvious that these conclusions are a gross oversimplification of conditions in the real world. Here, we see the difficulties faced by researchers in separating out the relative magnitude of effects of intrinsic and extrinsic factors in defining circadian rhythms of motor performance. In this case, for example, the ambient temperature will probably be considerably lower in the morning, which might far outweigh the influence of circadian variations in core temperature. And, just to further complicate matters, a circadian rhythm also exists in the sensitivity of the hypothalamus to changes in core temperature. As core temperature rises, the magnitude of its response in turning on cooling mechanisms (sweating rate, cutaneous vasodilatation) varies over the course of 24 hours. Such responses are greater during waking hours than during sleep. They are also more pronounced during peak exercise than at trough times of circadian fluctuations in core temperature. There exists evidence, too, that changes in environmental temperature can alter both the periodicity and amplitude of circadian rhythms. Confused yet?

Anyway, it will be interesting to see how this all pans out in the section of this chapter that examines the results of studies evaluating circadian rhythms in actual sports performance. Is the daily swing in core temperature a central factor for defining similar circadian variations in sports performance? Or do temporal changes in performance listen to other physiological clocks? How critical are circadian changes in body temperature to strategies for optimizing athletic success?

Muscle Strength

The data regarding circadian rhythms in force of muscle contraction are generally much more straightforward, being less affected by extrinsic factors. Reilly and colleagues reviewed seven studies that examined isometric strength (grip, back strength, leg extension) or dynamic-isokinetic knee strength in relation to different times of the day.[5] Consistently, these reports indicated that peak strength was exhibited between 5:00 and 7:00 p.m. (corresponding to peaks in core temperature) and that the amplitude was more than trivial (ranging from 4 to 10% of the average value).

A report by Nicolas and colleagues provided a somewhat different view of this issue. In this study, 12 adult males performed a series of 50 maximal contractions of the knee extensor muscles at a constant angular velocity (2.09 radians per second) at 6:00 a.m and again at 6:00 p.m. Expected maximal torque values were 7.7% greater at the later time. However, the rate of decline of strength with repeated contractions (that is, greater fatigue) was observed in the evening. So, by the time the subjects had achieved 20 repetitions, torque values were similar for the two testing times.[6]

Maximal Aerobic Power

The athlete's ability to utilize oxygen is critical to aerobic endurance performance. As measured during laboratory exercise testing, the maximal aerobic power ($\dot{V}O_2$max) is a composite expression of a myriad of physiological factors that define oxygen transport and uptake. Each has its own intrinsic biological rhythm.

One's oxygen uptake at rest (reflecting the basal metabolic rate) demonstrates clear-cut circadian rhythmicity, with the lowest levels at 4:00 a.m. and a peak in the late afternoon and early evening. At first thought, the coincidence of this peak with that of core body temperature might be expected, since metabolic rate normally responds to elevations in temperature by the Q_{10} effect (rise in metabolic rate by 10% for every 1 degree C rise in body temperature). However, Reilly pointed out that circadian variations in body temperature account for only 37% of those in resting $\dot{V}O_2$.

During exercise, things get a bit more complicated. For example, Reilly found that when studying a single subject, $\dot{V}O_2$ expressed as ml/kg/min while cycling at 150 watts peaked at 2:40 in the afternoon. However, with closer analysis, it was apparent that this variability was entirely due to circadian changes in body mass (the size-normalizing denominator) instead of $\dot{V}O_2$. But then, absolute $\dot{V}O_2$ was found to exhibit periodicity at lower work rates.

Identification of diurnal rhythms of $\dot{V}O_2$ during submaximal exercise may depend on the exercise model being employed. Some have found no periodicity to $\dot{V}O_2$ during submaximal work while others have, with a peak between 2:00 and 5:00 in the afternoon, found an amplitude of 13%.

No circadian variability has been observed in $\dot{V}O_2$max. However, as Reilly and colleagues pointed out in their book, this is a particularly difficult question to sort out. Variations in test-retest $\dot{V}O_2$max are influenced by subject motivation as well as variability of equipment measurement. These variations might well mask true endogenous biological rhythms in maximal aerobic power. If such intrinsic rhythms exist in maximal aerobic power, they are presumably of small amplitude. Reilly and colleagues noted that the amplitude of the circadian rhythmicity of $\dot{V}O_2$ at maximal exercise, if reflecting that at rest, would be about 0.5%. (Who knows, however, the extent that even such small, circadian rhythmic changes in physiological aerobic fitness might have on aerobic endurance performance where seconds count?)

Flexibility

Circadian variability has been reported in flexibility of certain joints (lumbar flexion and extension, lateral glenohumeral rotation, whole-body forward flexion) with amplitudes approaching 20% of the average daily level. Demonstrated times of peak flexibility in these rhythms vary considerably between subjects, but typically occur in the afternoon and evening hours.

Anaerobic Power

Performance on a 30-second all-out Wingate cycling test provides information regarding peak and mean anaerobic power. These variables demonstrate circadian rhythmicity, with highest values between 3:00 and 9:00 p.m. and an amplitude of 8%. Similar diurnal periodicity has been observed with bench exercises as well as with stair-running and jumping tests.

Hormones

Blood levels of a number of hormones that may have a bearing on sports performance demonstrate phasic circadian changes. Catecholamines (epinephrine and norepinephrine) reach their greatest values in the early afternoon. Deschenes and colleagues found rhythmicity in plasma lactate and norepinephrine responses to maximal exercise, with a nadir at 8:00 in the morning. Cyclical patterns of levels of cortisol and growth hormone, on the other hand, peak during the sleeping hours.

Psychological and Psychomotor Factors

Investigators have utilized a number of tools to examine circadian changes in mental alertness and arousal, which obviously are critical to success in many sports. Generally, they have found that these markers of mental function demonstrate circadian variability with peak levels in the afternoon. A high level of arousal may, however, be antithetical to performance in activities requiring fine-motor control. Tasks requiring hand steadiness and the ability to balance are more successfully accomplished in the morning.

Rating of perceived exertion (RPE), which places a numerical value to subjective feelings of fatigue during exercise, is said to demonstrate circadian rhythmicity with lowest levels (best psychological tolerance for exercise) in the late afternoon and early evening. It is difficult, however, to sort out whether cyclical changes in perception of effort reflect circadian variability of the physiological responses that trigger such feelings (heart rate, ventilation, metabolic rate), or whether independent, intrinsic biological variations in the central nervous system functions make us feel fatigued.

Reaction time to auditory or visual stimuli is greatest in the early evening hours, coinciding with the time of peak core temperature. As noted previously, this may reflect the direct effect of increased velocity of nerve conduction from a rise in body temperature. It is interesting, though, that faster reactions are apparently gained at the expense of accuracy, which is worse in the early evening.

How about temporal changes in the ability to strategize? No one knows, but processes like the ability to perform arithmetic and short-term memory are optimized in the early morning hours. Long-term memory may be different. One study found that school children's memory recall was 8% greater one week after material was presented to them at 3:00 p.m. than at 9:00 a.m. In general, circadian rhythms of cognitive processes tend to peak earlier in the day than those of physiological variables. And, interestingly, the circadian rhythms in mental tasks requiring a high degree of memory load peak 8 hours earlier. They also have a lower amplitude than those involving less memory work.

Self-rated feelings of mood and well-being tend to be accentuated midafternoon, around 2:00. Somewhat surprisingly, circadian rhythms in such measures have been found to be only minimally influenced by whether you are a morning or night person. Temperature peak is separated by about an hour in the two groups. Morning people have higher epinephrine levels at dawn, and their mood rhythms are shifted a couple of hours. But the basic circadian rhythms are similar for both groups.

Implications for Sport Performance

So much for the components of motor activity. With all these documented circadian rhythms—some with rather substantial amplitude—we might expect that similar periodicity would be observed in actual athletic performance. Let's look at the findings in the limited number of available studies. These investigations represent a large variety of research models (each with unique strengths and weaknesses), and most have simply compared performance at selected times of day rather than over the course of 24 hours. So, they really should be interpreted as time-of-day studies rather than as investigations examining circadian rhythms. But that's really alright, since athletic competitions don't typically occur in the wee hours of the morning.

Football (Soccer)

When a group of British footballers attempted to set an aerobic endurance record for five-a-side competition by playing continuously for four days, Reilly and Walsh saw an opportunity. Here was a chance to examine true 24-hour circadian variability in sports play. They measured the players' pace of activity with motion analysis and found a circadian rhythm with a peak at about 6:00 p.m. and a trough between 5:00 and 6:00 a.m. That was, at least, up until the 91st hour of play, when the participants began to have visual hallucinations and "transient schizoid behavior" from sleep deprivation, and the refs called the match off. A negative correlation was observed between activity levels and players' (not the authors') subjective feelings of fatigue.[7]

Swimming

Swimmers competing the 100-meter distance have been found to perform better at 5:00 p.m. than at 7:00 a.m. One study indicated best performances (by 3.6 and 1.9%, respectively) were observed in the evening in both the 400-meter crawl and repeated 50-meter trials.

Cycling

Young cyclists have provided better times in 16K races that were conducted in the afternoon, compared to those in the morning. The pedaling rate and velocity spontaneously selected by cyclists also varies over the course of a day. In the laboratory, Deschenes and colleagues could find no relationship between aerobic endurance time during a progressive cycling test to exhaustion and time of day in fit college students. Cycling sprinting power, as demonstrated by ergometers, is greater in the evening (5:00 to 7:00 p.m.) than in the morning hours (7:00 to 9:00 a.m.).

However, in that study, when repeating such a sprint five times, the rate of decay in performance was faster in the evening. And, when all was averaged out, the total work on the five trials was independent of time of day. This pattern resembles that previously noted for repeated measures of isokinetic strength.

Running

Marathon performance is closely linked to ambient temperature. Thus, it is not surprising that the best times are generally recorded in races conducted in the early morning. In this case, an extrinsic, environmental factor clearly masks any possible intrinsic, biological one.

Nationally ranked male competitors have reported their fastest 80-meter sprint times at 7:00 in the evening. Except for a small dip in the early afternoon, performance on multiple trials gradually improved during the course of the day.

Racket Sports

Serve velocity of tennis players is greater at 6:00 p.m. than at 9:00 a.m. However, the inverse has been observed in serving accuracy, which is optimal in the morning. Similar findings have been described with badminton players.

Mixed Sports

In one report, evening performance was superior in most swimmers, runners, and shot putters, and for a crew of runners. Reilly and colleagues noted that during track-and-field competition in the last half-century, world records in only the men's shot put and women's javelin have been set in the morning. These authors also highlighted the fact that middle-distance running records set by their British countrymen (Sebastian Coe, Steve Cram, Steve Ovett, and Dave Moorcroft) in the 1980s were all achieved after tea time (between 5:00 and 11:00 p.m.), acknowledging that few 1,500-meter events are actually scheduled in the morning hours.

Intrinsic Circadian Rhythms of Performance

Youngstedt and O'Connor argued that the changes in performance during the course of the day (outlined in the preceding section) were just as likely due to environmental and behavioral factors as to the dictates of an intrinsic biological clock.[8] Timing of meals, for instance, could alter glycogen stores. (It has been shown, in fact, that alterations in meal times can shift time of peak sprinting ability to later in the afternoon.) Some have claimed that coffee intake or, conversely, caffeine withdrawal can also affect periodicity of performance. Poorer performance in the morning might reflect sleep effects, particularly in joint stiffness. Other extrinsic factors to be considered are differing periods of precompetition rest, daily changes in ambient temperature, depressed morning levels of motivation, and scheduling of competitions.

Drust and colleagues directly rebutted these arguments, contending that abundant evidence indicates that diurnal periodicity in sports performance is an expression of endogenous biological rhythms. They note that many of the extrinsic factors postulated by Youngstedt and O'Connor, when cyclical changes of physiological function and performance persist, have been controlled in the laboratory setting.

To figure this out, it would be helpful to do a study to see if diurnal patterns of athletic performance continue to be evident in a constant routine condition (fixed light exposure, diet, and so on). Unfortunately, this would require playing soccer in a cave for 24 hours with a mandatory hourly intake of sports drink and chocolate bars. Therefore,

In the Midnight Hour

If you want to learn firsthand about circadian rhythms and performance, you should head to Fairbanks, Alaska, on June 21. Just tell your spouse, parents, or significant other that you're going out for milk, and go.

June 21st. In case you've forgotten, that's the date of the summer solstice, when the sun annually reaches the highest point in its arc across the sky in the Northern Hemisphere. In Alaska, the solar globe dips below the horizon for a short time, but it remains light all night long. This celestial event has been marked by mystics for centuries. Every year in Fairbanks since 1906, they've done it by playing baseball in the Midnight Sun Game. The local semipro team, the Goldpanners, hosts a team from elsewhere in the lower 48 states. The game starts at 10:30 at night and finishes around 1:30 the next morning. They never use artificial lighting, and the game has never been called for darkness. At midnight the game stops, and somebody traditionally sings the Alaska flag song.

How does the fact that the players' circadian clocks are a bit off-kilter affect the quality of the game? It's hard to tell for sure, but in terms of pure excitement, these games have been hard to top (a nifty pun, considering the competition takes place a mere 160 miles [260 km] from the Arctic Circle). In fact, in three straight years between 2000 and 2002, the game was decided by the Goldpanners in their final time at bat.

For equal drama, take the 1965 game. (A newcomer named Tom Seaver had started on the mound for the Goldpanners but had suffered a cut while trying to make a bare-handed grab of a short hopper in the fifth inning. He had to spend the rest of the game in the hospital emergency room.) It was the ninth inning, the Goldpanners led 4-3, and the Trojans of the University of Southern California were up. The bases were loaded, two were out, and the count was 3-2 on the batter Ken Walker. Two foul balls. Then—crack!—a powerful drive towards the left field wall. Which, with (or thanks to) a relieved gasp from the 2,500 frenzied hometown fans, curved foul. Muggs Mies went into his stretch, delivered the decisive curve ball, and struck Walker out! One can only suspect a Hollywood scriptwriter.

such an investigation has not been done. The closest is the study noted previously by Reilly and Walsh of soccer competitors in constant play for four days and nights, while rhythms of activity, RPE, and heart rate persisted. (The difficulties of performing such studies is highlighted in this report. Meaningful activity was lost in the fourth day due to "recurring instances of behavioral abnormalities.")

Perhaps with Solomon-like wisdom, Drust and colleagues had the best answer:

"Instead of considering that the circadian rhythms of sports performance are wholly exogenous in origin, an alternative explanation would be to consider that the complex changes required for exercise have both exogenous and endogenous components, and that the endogenous component is a reflection of the body clock. This implies that the circadian response to exercise is similar in origin to the rhythm of core temperature, and this could account for the general parallelism between the two rhythms."[8]

Implications for Athletes

Just how important or useful to the competitive athlete is this whole concept of diurnal rhythmicity of physiological function and performance? I suppose it depends on how one looks at it. Certainly, documentation is clear that peak performance in many sports events involving muscular power occurs in the late afternoon and early evening. Other data suggest that when mental acumen and fine motor function are important, morning or early afternoon is best. The amplitude of swings in function over the course of a day are appreciable, and could reasonably be expected to bear importance for performance, particularly in sports events in which very minor differences separate out the winner from the also-ran.

Drust and colleagues thought this way. The current research data, they said, "makes an understanding of the circadian variation in sports performance an important practical consideration for both athletes and coaches in competition and might have important implications for both the short- and long-term success of an athlete or team."[8]

On the other hand, a number of issues, considered collectively, suggests that all this information is, although very interesting, of limited practical value to the competing athlete.

1. Athletes and coaches rarely, if ever, have much of a say in the scheduling of athletic events. Spectator sports are arranged around times when people can come and watch, or are dictated by television scheduling. At the U.S. Open, depending on weather and duration of matches, tennis competition can begin early in the morning or much later, even approaching midnight.

2. Circadian rhythms affect all the competitors, not just you. Your opponents at the starting line are just as likely to gain from a 6:00 p.m. firing of the gun.

3. There is probably considerable variability among athletes for peak times of performance, which cannot be easily defined for any particular person.

4. Even if significant improvements in performance could be expected at certain times, environmental influences might well wash out the advantage. Like the wind picking up to 20 mph just before the afternoon javelin throw. I know if I need to be mentally sharp for a particular task, a tall latte will do it. Too, we're all well aware of dramatic fluctuations in performance that seem to come out of the blue for no obvious reason. The qualifier who knocks out the defending Wimbledon champ in the first round. The football team, trailing 23-0 after a disastrous first half, that comes out of the locker room looking like another team and rallies to win. All of these influences might negate biological-based circadian variations in performance.

It would be of great interest to athletes, on the other hand, if circadian rhythms could be demonstrated for effects of sports training. Picking the best time of day to practice, with the expectation of greatest performance improvement—now, that would be useful. (Keep in mind that improvements in performance from training result from adaptations to the stresses imposed by an exercise bout. So, we could be talking about circadian rhythms of the level of stress imposed by an afternoon's training run, or the magnitude of the body's aerobic physiological responses.)

We have little data to go on to see if daily periodicity of training responses actually occurs. Torii and colleagues reported that increases in estimated $\dot{V}O_2$max were greater when subjects trained for four weeks in the afternoon (between 3:00 and 3:30 p.m.), compared to those training in the morning or evening. (All subjects were tested in the afternoon.) Hill and colleagues reported that improvements in aerobic endurance time for a high-intensity work load (2.6 W/kg) in the morning was greater than in the afternoon in a small group of subjects ($N = 6$) who trained in morning. The opposite was true for those who trained in the afternoon. This suggested that training-induced performance might be predicted to occur optimally at the same time of day as the training. In another study, however, Hill and colleagues were unable to detect any circadian variations to training-induced improvements in $\dot{V}O_2$max. They did show, though, that for subjects who trained in the morning, values of ventilatory thresholds were higher after training. Those who trained in the afternoon demonstrated greater ventilatory thresholds when tested in the afternoon.[9]

Hildebrandt and colleagues described a 20% greater increase in muscle strength when subjects trained at 7:00 p.m. than at 9:00 a.m. In that study, as Reilly and colleagues pointed out, subjects were only tested at the time they trained.

These meager data provide just an inkling that there might be something to this idea of a best time of day for optimizing training effects.

Athletes would be most interested if there were. Here's something concrete, like diet and equipment, that they could readily control. Clearly, a great deal of research work needs to be done before any conclusions on the matter can be drawn.

Seasonal Rhythmicity in Performance

So far, we've been considering rhythmic changes in physiological factors and sports performance that vary in a circadian, or diurnal, fashion. What about patterns of change that fluctuate over a year's time, or with the seasons? Certainly, many examples of biological circannual rhythms exist among animals (hibernation, mating, migration). In humans, biological and environmental factors may combine to cause seasonal patterns in myocardial infarctions, asthma, mood, weekly energy expenditure, and body composition. Do these kinds of longer phasic changes occur in sports performance?

You can already see the problem in trying to answer this question. Many sports are performed only at particular times of the year, either by dictates of climate or custom, which presumably have nothing to do with intrinsic biological clocks. [A researcher from outer space landing on Earth might well conclude that annual biological rhythms must exist for football (coincidentally and maybe causally related to the falling of leaves), baseball (with a peak in the summer corresponding to beer consumption), and skiing (peak at times of children's winter school vacations).] Even in sports that are performed year-round, training regimens are periodized by athletes in order to peak for major competitions. These extrinsic factors are just too prominent to permit insights into any true biological circannual rhythms.

That's what Atkinson and Drust concluded in their review of seasonal rhythms and exercise.[10] They cite a couple of studies. Members of a British road-cycling team had a higher $\dot{V}O_2$max during a competitive season. Elite-level Dutch speed skaters demonstrated no seasonal changes in $\dot{V}O_2$max or performance on a Wingate anaerobic test. The bottom line is that seasonal changes in sports performance can usually be explained by extrinsic patterns of climate or training intensity. At present, no evidence exists of any meaningful influences of intrinsic circannual rhythms on sports performance.

Jet Lag and Performance

The evidence of the traditional argument for the strength of intrinsic biological rhythms becomes painfully clear when such rhythms are disturbed. This happens when you are transported rapidly over multiple time zones on the planet. Circadian rhythms are entrained principally to 24-hour cycles of light and dark. If your 747 takes off from JFK in New York at 8:00 on a winter evening, your biological clock (with its created physiological rhythms) is expecting that the dark portion of the cycle will be completed in about 12 hours. To its great surprise, however, it instead encounters light just six hours later as you touch down at Charles de Gaulle airport outside of Paris.

Such disturbances of circadian rhythms produce what we know, of course, as *jet lag*, that temporary but particularly unpleasant set of sensations that are experienced by almost all international travelers. Its symptoms include fatigue, poor sleep, decline in mental acumen, gastrointestinal upset, irritability (particularly, from personal experience, with one's spouse and children), headaches, and even mental confusion. Not exactly the way you'd want to spend your first day in Paris.

Although its mechanism remains to be clarified, there are some really interesting things about jet lag. Symptoms are worse when you're flying from west to east than the reverse. The more time zones you cross, the worse you'll feel. It is said that for each time zone you cross, you should add another day to fully recover. If you're young (pick your own definition) and in good physical shape, the effects will be less. In general, females probably experience more jet lag than males. Personality types seem to influence the magnitude of jet lag symptoms. If you're an extrovert or a night person, for example, you are likely to adapt more quickly to perturbations in biological rhythms. If you're highly neurotic, be prepared to suffer more. And if you stay in your hotel room after arriving rather than touring Notre Dame, the duration of your symptoms may well be extended.

It's not unreasonable to expect that jet lag with overseas travel would impair both physical and mental performance in a competitive sports situation. Athletes participating in international events have thus had great interest in the possible negative effects on physiology and performance of what has been termed *circadian adversity*. More importantly, they'd like to know how to avoid them. Surprisingly, the research literature regarding the effects of jet lag for athletic performance is not considerable. Among the few studies that have been conducted, many suffer from significant weaknesses in design. Consequently, uncertainty persists about the effects that disturbed biological circadian rhythms, per se, have on sports performance following international travel. Here is some of the research information we do have.

Wright and colleagues described what happened to physiological function and exercise performance of 97 male soldiers when they were transferred from Fort Hood, Texas, to a military base in Germany, a translocation of six time zones. Testing was performed during five days prior to their departure and repeated during the first five days of arrival, beginning eight hours after their plane landed. A majority of the soldiers described typical jet-lag symptoms of fatigue, weakness, headache, disturbed sleep, and irritability. These substantially diminished by the fifth day. Despite these complaints, maximal oxygen uptake, running economy, and RPE during treadmill testing were unchanged, as were measures of isometric strength. However, a decline in dynamic strength and muscular endurance of elbow flexors was observed. Similarly, performance on a 270-meter sprint deteriorated between 8 and 12% (figure 4.3).

Hill and colleagues reported that peak anaerobic power and 30-second anaerobic work capacity on a Wingate cycling test were reduced when a group of nonathletic subjects traveled from North America to France. The trip failed to affect grip strength, however.

A number of studies have attempted to assess differences in performance of athletic teams after long-distance travel to competitions.

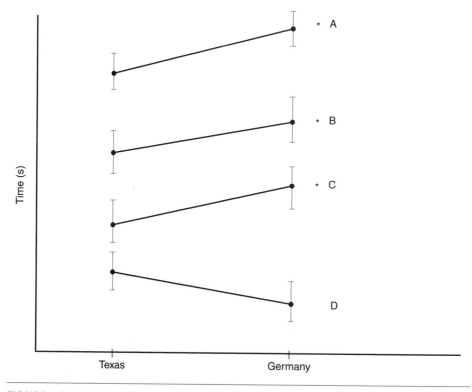

FIGURE 4.3. Effect of jet lag on performance: Line A is for a 2.8-kilometer run, line B is for a 270-meter sprint, line C is for a 100-meter fireman carry, and line D is for a 6-meter rope climb (76). * = $p < 0.05$.

For example, among 8,495 games in the National Basketball Association, visiting teams that traveled from the west coast to the east coast of the United States were found to have scored four points a game better than teams flying in the opposite direction. (However, other explanations for this observation might exist rather than the directional differences in jet lag. Perhaps the teams on the west coast are simply better than those from the east.) In another study, win-loss records were examined for National Football League teams between 1978 and 1987. It was found that the home-field advantage rose with increasing distance traveled by the visiting team.

Although it is generally assumed that long-distance travel across numerous time zones will result in a deterioration of athletic performance on arrival, a number of authors have not been convinced. On reviewing the experimental data, O'Connor and Morgan concluded that "no evidence exists in support of the view that rapid traversal of multiple time zones has an influence on athletic performance."[11] Youngstedt and O'Connor agreed, claiming that "the scientific evidence supporting the assumption [that air travel has detrimental effects on athletic performance] is neither consistent nor compelling."[8] Even if such decrements were to be documented, these detractors note that other factors during long-distance travel, such as disturbances in sleep cycles, fatigue, boredom, dehydration, and change in dietary patterns, might be just as likely to cause declines in performance as the desynchronization of biological circadian rhythms.

Equally uncertain is the efficacy of the many preventive measures and remedies that have been utilized by international travelers in the hope of avoiding jet lag. These have included dietary intake plans (high-protein breakfasts, high-carbohydrate dinners), gradually changing sleep patterns before traveling, exercise, light exposure, hydration, sleeping pills, alcohol, and supplemental melatonin. And if the American athlete is flying to Singapore, the advice would be to go through Hawaii rather than London (travelling from east to west is best). The most sound advice, however, remains to fly early enough to permit dissipation of jet-lag symptoms before the start of competition.

Latitudinal Jet Lag

The preceding discussion has focused on what happens when you cross time zones and make large hops of longitude by traveling east to west or vice versa. But what happens if you take a long trip north or south, crossing latitude lines, maybe without even leaving the same time zone? This, in fact, might be expected to disturb circadian rhythms in another manner. Diurnal biological rhythms are entrained to light-dark cycles, but such phases of light and dark vary dramatically as you move from the equator toward the poles. If you fly on June 21 from Central America, where the light-dark ratio during 24 hours is about 12:12, to Greenland, you will find the ratio has changed to almost 24:0.

The circadian clock adjusts for such changes in the light-dark cycle (as it must do during the changes of seasons throughout the year in a single location). You might expect, however, that for a brief period after you land, your physiological rhythms will be in a bit of disarray and your capacity for physical performance might suffer. The effect of sudden marked latitudinal displacement on athletic performance, however, has not been determined.

Melatonin

No discussion of circadian rhythms, jet lag, and sports performance would be complete without a mention of melatonin, which may serve as the mediator by which the biological clock in the suprachiasmatic nucleus (SCN) is linked to light-dark cycles. Melatonin is secreted by the pineal gland in a diurnal fashion that is very strongly influenced by light. Levels during the dark of night can be 30 times greater than in the daytime. And the SCN is equipped with melatonin receptors, presumably to stay in tune with light-dark cycles.

What happens to blood-melatonin levels when you exercise? The reports have been conflicting. One study found that that plasma-melatonin levels in adult females rose transiently at least twofold after 60 minutes of exercise. This is similar to previous findings in men. But others have described either a decline in melatonin concentration 3 hours after 20 minutes of exercise, or no changes in blood-melatonin levels at all after sessions of exercise.

It should be recognized that these reports describe different forms of exercise performed at various times in the day-night cycle, with levels drawn at different times postexercise. The true response of plasma-melatonin levels to physical exercise remains to be clarified.

On the other hand, melatonin has a number of physiological effects that seem rather incontrovertible (and of some interest to athletes), including the following:

- Lower body temperature (hypothermic effect)
- A sedative or hypnotic effect
- Alleviation of symptoms of jet lag, perhaps by speeding the resetting of circadian rhythms after long-distance travel (This effect is somewhat less definite.)

From these influences, one might immediately suspect that administration of melatonin might offer some real advantages to the athlete in promoting exercise performance. For instance, a reduction in body temperature would be expected to permit greater aerobic endurance when competing in hot ambient conditions. And alleviation of jet-leg symptoms could reduce any decline in motor performance after international travel. But, alas, the experimental data addressing these issues is disappointing. It doesn't seem to work, at least in respect to reduction of hyperthermia with exercise. And taking melatonin before some kinds of athletic events might even be detrimental to performance.

Atkinson and colleagues provided a table outlining 17 studies that have demonstrated a hypothermic effect of administered melatonin, with a reduction in core body temperature ranging from 0.01 to 0.3 degrees C.[12] Interestingly, although the diurnal periodicity of melatonin secretion from the pineal gland (highest in the night) is the mirror image of that of core temperature, no one has been able to verify a causal relationship between the two. This hypothermic effect of melatonin, however, has not been observed to translate into any improvement of exercise tolerance in hot ambient conditions.

In its hypnotic qualities, melatonin has been documented to slow the subject's visual reaction time as well as reduce alertness. But if you are a rat, here's good news. Melatonin can be expected to improve your short-term memory (exactly for what is uncertain). Unfortunately, if you are a human, no similar effect has been observed. In fact, in performance tests, melatonin has been observed to decrease short-term memory, as well as balance and proprioception. The influences would not seem to bode well for certain kinds of sports performance. Atkinson and colleagues noted, though, that if you were to take melatonin in the evening to promote sleep, any negative effects on cognitive performance should disappear by the following morning. The bottom line is, though, that despite certain hypothetical advantages, there is no reason to expect that administration of melatonin for its hypothermic or hypnotic effects will enhance athletic performance.

Melatonin may have a role in preventing jet lag, however. If these symptoms of travel-induced disturbances of circadian rhythms truly do deteriorate sports performance, it is a possible remedy. A number of extensive reviews have examined the published research literature regarding the ability of melatonin to reduce jet lag. The general conclusion is that it often works, at least to some extent. Just how is unknown. It could be a result of its sedative effect or it might be a matter of shifting circadian rhythms.

Would taking melatonin help an athlete flying over the Atlantic Ocean to participate in a track and field meet in London prevent symptoms of jet lag, blocking any impairment of performance the next day? That's a key question. The simple answer is that no one knows. To my knowledge, the question has never been addressed experimentally. But there is one report in soldiers, who serve as a reasonable surrogate.

Lagarde and colleagues assessed changes in both static and dynamic exercise performance for U.S. Air Force reservists on a flight from San Antonio, Texas, to an air base in Landes, France. Nine subjects took 5 milligrams of melatonin one day before the flight, again during the flight, and also during the first three days after landing. Another group took a placebo. On testing hand-grip strength before and after travel, the placebo group demonstrated a decrement in performance during the initial three days in France, while no decline was seen in those taking melatonin. The trip did not affect performance of either squat jumps or multiple jumps in either group. So, in this study, melatonin seemed to reduce the negative effect of jet lag on static movement, but not dynamic exercise.

Despite its potential usefulness, there seems to be general cautiousness about taking melatonin to alleviate jet lag symptoms. Proper timing and dosage have not been completely determined. Although taking melatonin has generally been considered safe, without acute side effects, long-term toxicology studies have not been performed. For those interested in preventing decrements in sports performance after long-distance travel, such discretion may be particularly warranted.

The Athlete and Jet Lag

So what does all this mean for the athlete traveling long distances for international competition? In 2004, having reviewed most of the material you've just read, the FIMS (Federation Internationale de Médecine du Sport) issued an official position statement titled "Air Travel and Performance in Sports." Their conclusion? "Although some athletes, anecdotally, report impaired performance after air travel, there is no consistent or compelling evidence showing that either air travel across multiple time zones or jet lag symptoms cause a reduction in sports performance."[13]

Just in case you're one of those anecdotal few, however, the document outlines a number of practical strategies that athletes might consider in order to alleviate or prevent symptoms of jet lag. These include exposure to bright light (which reportedly creates shifts of biological phases), melatonin (which shifts the biological clock in the opposite direction as bright light), and exercise (which acts like melatonin). Refer to this source for the details, which are numerous, as to the most effective timing of these interventions (www.fims.org). Be careful, though. If you err on the proper timing, you might only make things worse.

So notes the FIMS disclaimer: "It cannot be overemphasized that these three methods for shifting circadian rhythms depend critically on the timing of the intervention. Ill-timed bright light, exercise, or melatonin could plausibly exacerbate jet-lag symptoms or delay resynchronization beyond the time it usually takes to adapt to a new time zone." I was not able to find in this position statement, though, the seemingly best advice: Arrive at the destination early enough to allow symptoms of jet lag to subside before the day of competition.

Notes

1. Reiberg, A.E. et al.2001. "The birth of chronobiology: Julien Joseph Virey 1814." *Chronobiology International* 18: 173-186.
2. Read a fascinating first-person account of his two-month subterranean ordeal: Siffre, Michel. 1964. *Beyond time*. New York: McGraw Hill.
3. This book provides an impressive listing of just how markers of body function, disease, and biochemistry in the human body ebb and flow over the course of a day: Foster, R.G., and L. Kreitzman. 2004. *Rhythm of life*. New Haven, CT: Yale University Press.
4. This book is an excellent source of information on circadian rhythms: Dulap, C., J.J. Loros, and P.J. DeCoursey. 2004. *Chronobiology. Biological Timekeeping*. Sunderland, MA: Sinauer Associates.
5. Reilly, T., G. Atkinson, W. Gregson, J. Forsyth, B. Edwards, and J. Waterhouse. 2006. "Some chronological considerations related to physical exercise." *Clinical Therapy* 157: 249-264.
6. For more information on the effect of circadian rhythms on physiological variables, read the following sources: Deschennes, M.R., R.V. Sharma, K.T. Brittingham, D.J. Casa, L.E. Armstrong, and C.M. Marsh. 1998. "Chronobiological effects on exercise performance and selected physiological responses." *European Journal of Applied Physiology* 77: 249-256. Nicolas, A., A. Gauthier, N. Bessot, S. Moussay, and D. Davenne. 2005. "Time-of-day effects on myoelectric and mechanical properties of muscles during maximal and prolonged isokinetic exercise." *Chronobiology International* 22: 997-1011.
7. Reilly, T, and T. Walsh. 1981. "Physiological, psychological, and performance measures during an endurance record for 5-a-side soccer play." *British Journal of Sports Medicine* 15: 122-128.
8. Conflicting viewpoints of the effect of circadian rhythms on athletes can be found in the following: Drust B., J. Waterhouse, G. Atkinson, B. Edwards, and T. Reilly. 2005. "Circadian rhythms and sports performance—an update." *Chronobiology International* 22: 21-44. Youngstedt, S.D., and P.J. O'Conner. 1999. "The influence of air travel on athletic performance." *Sports Medicine* 28: 197-207.

9. References for circadian rhythm effects on training responses: Hill, D.W., J.A. Leiferman, N.A. Lynch, B.S. Dangelmaier, and S.E. Burt. 1998. "Temporal specificity in adaptation to high intensity exercise." *Medicine and Science in Sports and Exercise* 30: 450-455. Hildebrandt, G., C. Guttenbruner, C. Reinhart et al. 1990. "Circadian variation of isometric training in man." In *Chronobiology and chronomedicine Vol. II*, ed. E. Moran E, 322-329. Frankfurt: Peter Lang. Torii, J., S. Shinkai, S. Hino et al. 1993. "Effect of time of day on adaptive response to a 4-week aerobic exercise training program." *Journal of Sports Medicine and Physical Fitness* 32: 348-352.

10. Atkinson, G., and B. Drust. 2005. "Seasonal rhythms and exercise." *Clinics in Sports Medicine* 24: e25-e34.

11. Additional reading on jet lag and athletic performance: O'Connor, P.J., and W.P. Morgan. 1990. "Athletic performance following rapid traversal of multiple time zones." *Sports Medicine* 10: 20-30.

12. Atkinson, G., B. Drust, T. Reilly, and J. Waterhouse. 2003. "The relevance of melatonin to sports medicine and science." *Sports Medicine* 33: 809-831.

13. O'Connor, P.J., S.D. Youngstedt, O.M. Buxton, and J. Breus. 2004. "FIMS Position statement." *Air Travel and Performance in Sports.* www.fims.org.

TAKE-HOME MESSAGES

1. Regular phasic changes in biological function are an inherent quality of all living beings. These oscillations, which are usually diurnal or circadian, include variables that influence athletic performance.

2. The extent that circadian rhythms in physiological and psychological variables truly affect athletic performance and responses to training remains uncertain. Particularly, it is not clear whether the magnitude of such effects outweighs those of extrinsic or environmental factors.

3. Although they are not well documented, it is reasonable to expect that interruptions in circadian rhythms, as manifested by symptoms of jet lag, may transiently negatively affect athletic performance after long-distance travel.

CHAPTER 5

Timing is everything: In making shots, in making love, in making dinner.

J. Gibbon and C. Malapani[1]

IT'S ALL IN THE TIMING

Keeping Your Eye on the Ball

You're just settling in at your favorite restaurant, Chez Nous. The waiter has taken your order, the usual bœuf en daube, to be washed down with an exquisite '96 Côtes du Rhône. In anticipation of your meal, you gaze around the restaurant. The milieu is warm and comfortable, the other diners are chatting amiably. The weather is superb for late autumn in New England, but it's expected to turn colder by the weekend. You review your day—not entirely unsuccessful. You accomplished a great deal, but the leaves still need raking.

By now, however, you're beginning to feel a bit of disquiet. It surely seems like it's taking them a long time with the dinner. The service here is usually excellent. After another period of considering your plans for tomorrow, you really do feel uncomfortable. And the people at the next table, who arrived after you, are already on their main course. A decision is made—you stop the waiter and inquire as to the reason for the delay. "Ah, monsieur, quel dommage," he explains. "I accidentally dropped your order on the floor leaving the kitchen. But, pas de problème, we're cooking you another!" Totally galled, you storm out of the restaurant, heading for a drive-through burger and fries.

What happened here? According to what is called *scalar expectancy theory*, as soon as the waiter first took your order, an internal clock, driven by the oscillatory activity of spontaneously firing nerve cells, began ticking in your brain. The ticks were stored up in an accumulator, which provided you with a sense of present or working time, what duration had elapsed since the order headed for the kitchen. Now, waiting for your dinner in this restaurant is an experience you've had many times before, and a memory of the previous time durations between ordering and receiving your meal is stored in your central nervous system. You matched up the accumulated working time with the past time durations, became aware of the discrepancy, and made a conscious decision to act based on differences, or the ratio, between the two.

How accurate were you? Repeated in a similar setting, you'd probably be very close. You became aware, upset, and acted, all in an appropriate time scale. But consider how this scenario might have changed if things were different. Suppose instead of dining alone, you were engaged in a scintillating conversation with a fascinating companion? Or, on the other hand, if you were pressed for time to make it to the theatre for an 8:00 curtain? The tempo of your clock, or at least your attention to it, would have been very different.

The previous scenario, which we've all experienced in one form or another, reminds us how an acute perception of time governs our daily activities and decisions. Indeed, it's difficult to think of any action that doesn't involve some kind of temporal sense.[1] We need to perceive our environment in both spatial and temporal realms. How long do you wait for the red light to change before realizing that it's malfunctioning and driving on through? How do you safely cross a busy street?

In animals, such processes are clearly linked to their survival value. You will no doubt recall from freshman biology class the African mormyrid fish, which creates an electrical field around its body to detect the motion and speed of other fish. This mechanism is effective for tracking and avoidance when it gets really dark down on the ocean floor. Or animals, like the barn owl, which can localize fleeing prey in the black of night by computing the difference in sound coming to one ear from that arriving at the other. (Think about this. Those animals with larger heads—a greater distance between the ears—should be able to discriminate such differences more easily than those with smaller heads.)

For athletes, the usual challenge is to identify a visual duration and match it to a motor activity. The tennis player must identify the course of the falling ball before striking a lob. The center on the basketball team can't allow himself to spend more than three seconds in the paint (the referee is counting the same duration). The football quarterback must judge the spot he should aim his pass based on (a) the time it will take for the receiver to reach that point and (b) the speed of the ball in the air. There are no watches to help make those decisions. They're all based on intrinsic timekeeping mechanisms. And, as we'll discuss, most aren't even in the realm of cognitive decision making. The astounding feats of sports performance we regularly witness from athletes are products of internal timekeepers that are matched tightly with finely tuned motor actions, well outside their conscious awareness.

This chapter examines some of the theories about how this all happens. It also considers whether time perceptions of athletes differ from those of nonathletes and if these temporomotor links can be improved with training.

Musicians Keeping Time

In the second movement of Bruckner's Seventh Symphony, there comes a point when a triangle roll is followed by a single crash of the cymbals. This is, in fact, the single note that this instrument performs in the entire symphony. Frank Wilson, in his article "Music and the Neurology of Time," cites Jens Rossel as describing that "this note becomes the occasion of indescribable anguish to almost every cymbal player responsible for its delivery. It must come at precisely the right instant, or it simply ruins everything. A few minutes before, you always see the fellow begin to turn in his chair, rub his hands, and wipe his palms on his trousers. When he stands up, he plants his feet, just so, like a baseball catcher bracing himself for a fast pitch. The moment comes and the cymbals crash. It's a matter of just a few milliseconds, but what it represents to the music is either life or death."[2]

Every performing musician has been there. In most musical settings, the precise matching of perception, time, and motor execution are critical. And the parallels of musical virtuosity—the remarkable ability to match timekeeping with muscular effort—with athletic performance have not been lost on scientific observers. Itzhak Perlman, flowing through the intricate passages of a Beethoven violin concerto, can rightly be considered an elite small-muscle athlete. Indeed, concluded the neurologist Frank Wilson, "the well-trained musician is, after all, an individual whose muscular prowess generally surpasses anything encountered on the athletic field."[2] (The virtuoso violinist lacks, of course, an opponent who is attempting with all his effort to inhibit such harmony, a game clock, and 85,000 screaming fans.)

Precise timing of coordinated finger movements in the production of notes is the essence of musical performance. The ability of instrumentalists to accomplish this at extraordinary speed (as in, say, a Paganini violin concerto) is a fundamental skill of accomplished musicians. Efforts of this author to enlighten the eager reader on exact speeds that music can be performed have been met with only partial success. The best I can do is report that on an autumn evening in 2003, an Italian named Carmelo Crucitti set the world's record for the most rapid playing by a bassoonist when he completed the Rimsky-Korsakov's "Flight of the Bumble Bee" in 33.8 seconds. That piece contains 791 notes, so Carmelo's internal clock, his intrinsic metronome as it were, was firing every 0.045 seconds, or 23 times a second. (One might expect the time would be even shorter if played on a violin or piano.)

Of course, we do not know how many mistakes he made. You might expect that the faster you play, the more errors you would make. But, interestingly, when it comes to timing accuracy, the same may hold true if you play slower. Talented pianists who play scales at different tempos have been found to be most accurate when they were playing 7 or 8 notes per second (intervals of 0.07 second). Diminished accuracy is observed at both faster and slower speeds. It has been pointed out that this particular frequency coincides with the preferred (and upper limit of) rate of alternations of flexion and extension across a single joint when performing an automatic movement (such as signing your name). The idea that these two observations might be physiologically related is an intriguing one.

Although Wilson noted that "even superficial reflection about this process impels one to the conclusion that the brain mechanisms involved must be of very high order and among the most complex found in biological systems,"[2] our understanding of the neurophysiological basis for musical skill remains vague. It has generally been assumed that these artists rely on an intrinsic clock that serves as an internal metronome, conducting coordinated muscle contractions. And, recognizing previous neurophysiological research, the basal ganglia and cerebellum are the parts of the brain that have been considered as key to the temporomotor coordination that underlies musical performance skills. Clearly, too, such mechanisms must be on automatic, since the milliseconds that separate closely spaced notes don't allow enough time for cognitive reflection.

Can you be born with the capacity to perform finely tuned sequences of notes necessary for musical performance? The question hasn't been truly resolved. Evidence indicates that the neuromuscular systems of those who have achieved musical success operate differently than yours and mine. To no one's surprise, skillful pianists are seen to possess motor and perceptual timing in laboratory testing that is superior to nonpianists. Musicians are also more accurate than nonmusicians in estimating time. But, then again, these talented people put in a lot more hours of practice than you or I do.

We'll return later to musicians as models of perceptuomotor timekeeping when we discuss the training of such abilities. You can guess that parallels between the acquisition of musical skill and catching ground balls at second base might be both expected and instructive.

It should be emphasized here that perfection of sensorimotor timing in the production of music is not really the artist's goal. If it were, we could simply have all music produced by a computer. In fact, musical performance is based on nuances of a piece that provide variation not only in the tempo but also in the shaping of notes, dynamics, intonation, and a host of factors that make each musician's performance unique. These are the differences that separate one musician or symphony orchestra from another, and the reason that we can listen to performances of Beethoven's Eroica Symphony over a lifetime without losing a sense of its freshness, beauty, and power.

Challenges of Perceptuomotor Timing in Sports

Athletes, of course, need to do more than simply estimate time intervals. Their task is to couple visual information with their perception of time, an accomplishment that is, in fact, often the very essence of athletic competition. Indeed, for a great many sports, it's the ability of players to track an object visually (ball, puck, shuttlecock), and then employ a timing device that enables them to initiate a motor act of particular direction, force, or duration at just the right moment.

Consider the player spiking the ball in volleyball, the wide receiver leaping over the defender in the end zone to catch a game-winning pass, the Liverpool goalkeeper diving for a save. Indeed, athletic success—being number one (not to mention the multimillion dollar contract)—goes to those who can best enact this scenario. In the end, it all basically just boils down to a neurophysiological battle.

What makes these responses even more amazing, of course, is that for the most part, they all occur beneath the level of conscious effort. They happen much too quickly for us to mull over how we might act, but, more importantly, they challenge the limits of time required for electrical activity in the neurons and muscular contractile apparatus that makes such feats possible. Let's look at a few examples.

Baseball

Hitting a pitched baseball has been regarded by some as the single most difficult challenge in all sports.[3] Consider this: The pitcher toes the rubber, winds up, and delivers a 70 to 100 mph fastball toward home plate, 60 feet away. There stands the batter, wielding a slab of lumber whose optimal point of contact with the ball is about 3 inches long. At the speed of the pitch, the time from the release of the ball to the hoped-for point of contact with the bat is about 450 milliseconds. During this time—a little less than half a second—the batter must do the following:

● Visually identify and track the oncoming ball
● Decide whether or not to swing
● Recognize the type of pitch (slider, fastball, knuckle ball)
● Time the coincidence of a complex motor act (swinging the bat) with the arrival of the ball across the plate

It takes 160 milliseconds from when the swing of the bat is initiated to when it meets the ball crossing the plate. Given a visuomotor reaction time (from seeing the ball to moving his muscles) of 200 milliseconds, the batter's decisions about swinging would be expected to occur 90 milliseconds after the pitcher delivers the ball. That's when the ball has traveled about 15 feet, one-quarter of its trip to the plate.

After the ball is released from the pitcher's hand, its trajectory in the sight line of the batter directly to center field changes little from 0 degrees until late in its pathway (that is, at the start, the ball is pretty much coming straight at the batter). The angle then rapidly reaches 90 degrees as the ball passes over the plate. As it does so, the angular velocity of the ball in the batter's sight is extraordinary—up to 500 degrees per second, which is much faster than the human eye can follow it (about 70 degrees per second).

Can baseball batters keep their eye on the ball? Or, more to the point, can they follow the ball with their eyes to the point of its contact with the bat? Robert Watts and Terry Bahill set out to find out. In the laboratory, they rigged batters with devices that measured eye movements as they swung at a simulated pitch (a white plastic ball threaded on a fishing line and propelled by a pulley). They had a number of interesting findings. First, a professional player was able to visually track the ball at an angular velocity in his vision up to 130 degrees per second. As noted previously, that's a lot faster than has been described in nonathletes. It would seem, at least based on this one subject, that the professional ball player has rather an astounding ability to visually track a pitched baseball as it nears the plate. That athlete could follow the ball to within 5.5 feet of home plate, but not after.

The authors then asked the question, how slow would the ball have to go so that the batter could actually keep his eye on it until contact with the bat? Keep in mind that it's not really a matter so much of the speed of the ball, but rather of its velocity when crossing the batter's field of vision. It's easy to visually track the ball during the first portions of the pitch, when the angular velocity in the batter's vision is very small—it's coming right at him. But the speed of the ball is actually greater at the beginning than when it crosses the plate. At that point, the angular velocity becomes too high for the batter to visually track the ball. That's why it can't be seen after it reaches about 6 feet in front of the plate.

Anyway, these investigators ran a computer simulation to try to address their question. Can a ball be pitched slowly enough so that a batter could watch it all the way to the plate? The computer's answer was never. They found that the slowest a pitch can be delivered and still reach the plate is 21 mph (34 kmph). Even at this lugubrious pace, the angular velocity as the ball crossed the plate would exceed human capacity for tracking.

Having said all this, one strategy would enable a batter to watch the ball closer to its contact with the bat. Watts and Bahill saw this in one of their subjects. Batters can visually track the pitched ball during the first portions of its flight, then jump their vision ahead (that's called a *saccade*) and then let the ball catch up to the focal point. Commented the authors, "If you want to see the ball hit the bat, you can make your anticipatory saccade early in the trajectory. This means you have to take your eye off the ball at precisely the time when you want to see the ball best. Using an anticipatory saccade to put your eye ahead of the ball may be an oft-trained strategy, but it is probably not the best strategy for hitting the ball."[3]

In fact, they wondered, why would a batter want to see the ball contact the bat? If you think about it, this wouldn't seem to be of much value. It would be too late at that point to change the direction of the swing of the bat. Given the required reaction time, that decision must come sooner, in anticipating or predicting the ball's path before it arrives.

Their final conclusion: "It has often been said that athletes are dumb. Our studies have shown the contrary. They are not paid a million dollars for their six-month job because of their bodies; it's because of their brains. The players that are paid the most have the best brains: They can predict the flight of the pitch better than other mere mortals can."[3]

Of course, too, the coincidence of swinging of the bat and the arrival of the ball must be exquisitely timed. As Adair noted, "if he swings as much as 1/100 of a second early, the ball will go down the left field line. If he is 1/100 of a second late, the ball will go foul into the stands down the right field line."[3]

But wait, there's more. Due to gravity, the ball falls in its trajectory toward the batter, which is magnified since the pitcher's mound is 10 inches higher than home plate. As the batter awaits the arrival of the pitch, the ball can descend as much as 3 meters. And, of course, the path of the ball, particularly late in the pitch, is open to all sorts of vagaries at the dictates of the wily pitcher. A knuckle ball wobbles in flight and can change direction more than once. A curve ball can move from a straight flight by as much as 0.4 meters. The slider curves away near the end of the pitch.

"The complexity of hitting," noted Stephen Kindel in an article in *Forbes* magazine, "is why baseball, of all sports, rewards relative failure so well. An NFL quarterback who hits his receiver less than 50% of the time or an NBA center who sinks fewer than half his baskets would soon be training as a stockbroker or selling beer. But baseball rewards .300 hitters—failure rates of 70%—with enormous contracts."[3]

All of the events that go into hitting a pitched baseball occur at a subconscious level. There's just not enough time to add an extra neural loop to the cerebral cortex, to think. But that's not to say that batters don't use cognitive processes to enhance their batting average. Ted Williams, arguably the best ever at this challenge, was a firm believer that proper thinking is 50% of effective hitting. He said, "You learn what you might expect in certain situations. Pitchers pick on your weaknesses, or what they fooled you with last time. But did I guess? Boy, I guess I did!"[4] (And good guessing it was, too. Good enough for a .344 lifetime batting average, three years at .400 or better).

There is both anecdotal and experimental evidence, in fact, that a batter's expectations, even before the ball leaves the pitcher's hand, is important for batting success. This could be, as Ted Williams emphasized, knowledge of a pitcher's tendencies, the pitch count, and past experience. Too, expert batters often appear to use particular visual clues, such as the release point during the pitcher's arm motion (compared to nonexperts, who fix on the pitcher's head and face).

Tennis

Now, I've never tried to hit a major-league fastball, but I did once attempt to return Andy Roddick's serve in the quarterfinals of the French Open. (Okay, so this was actually in a recent dream after an overindulgence at a friend's wedding.) Anyway, apparently to no one's amazement, I was leading 4-2 in the second set and was up 15-40 when Andy surprised me by firing one of his 138 mph (222 kmph) serves up the *T*. Since a distance of around 80 feet (24 m) separated the point where he struck the ball from the spot where I was cowering behind the baseline, I had fewer than 400 milliseconds to respond. Given the visuomotor reaction times previously noted, I had to recognize where the ball was going, track its flight, start to move my legs into position, and decide where and when to initiate my stroke, all pretty much just as the ball was leaving my opponent's racket (figure 5.1). One difference was for the better—I didn't have to swing at the ball. I simply had to block it back. And one for the worse—the ball was going to bounce (who knows where?). Knowing Andy, it was going to depart from its flight path after I'd lost sight of it, probably kicking up high and away. Fortunately, this is where I woke up.

Cricket

The batter in a cricket match faces time dilemmas similar to that of the returner of a tennis serve—tracking down and timing a swing at a rapidly approaching projectile that suddenly strikes earth and diverts at an unpredictable angle.[5] At Oxford University, Peter McLeod and Simon Jenkins analyzed the neuromuscular responses to striking a cricket ball and concluded, in fact, that the game might be—despite direct evidence to the contrary—totally impossible. In this sport, the batsman awaits a ball bowled at speeds up to 40 meters per second (m/s), or about 95 mph (150 kmph). The ball typically strikes the ground within 5 feet (1.5 m) of the batsman, slows to a speed of 25 to 30 meters per second, then bounces at a variable angle. Some quick

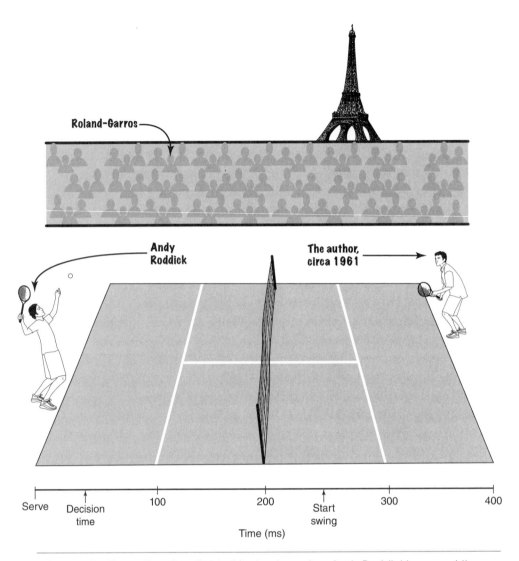

FIGURE 5.1. The author (in a flight of fantasy) receives Andy Roddick's serve at the French Open. By the expected times required for visuomotor reaction and movement of the racket, decision making would be required almost immediately after the ball left the server's racket.

arithmetic indicates that the batsman should not have sufficient time after the bounce for a normal reaction (200 milliseconds) that would allow him to accurately swing the bat. Yet skilled cricket players somehow accomplish this. In fact, they do this by timing the arrival of the ball within 3 milliseconds.

Table Tennis

Ditto. Except at point-blank range.

Athletes: Masters of Perceptuomotor Timing

Obviously, trained athletes are much more capable of performing these perceptuomotor timing tasks than average mortals are. How do they do it? Are their nervous systems and motor functions more finely tuned? Or do they take advantage of indirect cues that permit them to better anticipate the course of oncoming balls and pucks? The mystery remains incompletely solved, but it would seem that both answers are probably correct.

Although coaches and fans think of players as having a great arm or lightning-fast breakaway speed, researchers have more accurately considered athletes as experts at visuotemporal processing. In examining just what separates athletes' timing abilities from those of nonathletes, a number of factors have been considered, including the following:

- *Reaction time.* The duration required to detect a sensory stimulus and respond by initiating a motor act is a measure of the fundamental electrical properties within the nervous system. Obviously, for athletes, shorter is better. A fast reaction time gives a baseball batter more time to decide if, where, and when to swing the bat. He could then make his choice later in the ball's flight toward home plate when it was easier to tell just where the ball was headed.

- *Coincidental timing.* This is the ability to match a motor action with the arrival of an object. The third baseman must time his leap for a line drive at just the right instant when the ball arrives. To accomplish this, he must have some means of estimating the velocity of the ball.

- *Anticipation.* The ability to predict the location and flight of a pitched ball is very helpful. For instance, athletes may sense where the ball is going even as it is being thrown or hit.

Reaction Time

It could be that the electrical properties and conduction velocities of athletes' neurons are more enhanced than those of nonathletes. Traditionally, average reaction time in the laboratory setting (such as pushing a button in response to a flash of light) for human beings is about 200 milliseconds. Some investigators have suggested that it might be shorter. For instance, when D. Lee and coworkers had subjects jump up to hit balls that were falling from different heights, their reaction times varied between 55 and 130 milliseconds. A number of other studies have suggested that reaction to visual information can also be substantially shorter than 200 milliseconds. What's interesting, though, is that investigators have generally failed to find that such basic reaction times are any different in athletes than in untrained subjects. Moreover, these simple reactions times do not seem to improve with practice or sport training.[6]

At the same time, it might be suspected that athletes have superior reaction times in tasks that are specific to their sport. This idea has been supported by studies indicating that trained athletes in certain sports can more quickly respond when choosing between reactions to a stimulus. Termed a *go-no-go* reaction time, this is what baseball batters use when deciding whether or not to swing at a pitch. For those who are anatomically inclined, brain imaging studies have demonstrated that such decisions are made in the anterior cingulate cortex, with inhibitory control (discerning that the pitch is going to be in the dirt, for example) focused in the dorsolateral and ventral lateral prefrontal sites.

In one report, baseball players of varying levels of skill and experience and nonathletes were tested on their speed in deciding whether or not to press a key, depending on a color display that appeared on a computer screen. The choice reaction time was 16% shorter for the baseball players than for the nonathletes. Among the players, a negative relationship was observed between skill level and go-no-go time.

This study also showed that two years of baseball practice shortened choice reaction time. In addition, no difference was observed in go-no-go time between first-year baseball players and nonathletes. From these observations, the following suggestions were made:

- As opposed to simple reaction times, choice reactions are trainable.
- The shorter reaction times of trained athletes are not innate.

Similar findings about length of choice reaction times have been confirmed using similar testing procedures with fencers and basketball players. However, some have criticized the use of choice reaction times measured by this color-computer approach for identifying sport skill, given its generic nature.

Coincidental Timing

The ability to match the arrival of an object (say, a pitched ball) with a motor act (swinging at the ball) relies on an accurate means of estimating the object's incoming velocity. In most sports, as previously noted, the incoming object has very little angular velocity in the athlete's field of vision until just before it arrives (when that velocity suddenly becomes very fast). So, rate of image movement in the retina of the eye would not seem to be helpful in estimating velocity.

Instead, estimating the speed of the incoming object to permit coincidental timing is probably achieved by figuring out relative changes in the size of the object as it nears. That is, as the pitched ball approaches the batter, it gets larger in his field of vision. And the faster it comes, the more rapidly it expands. Let's raise the scientific sophistication of this discussion a bit by noting that the velocity (V) of the oncoming ball can be calculated as follows:

$$V = (D^2/s)(d\theta/dt)$$

In this equation, D is distance, s is the radius of the ball, and $d\theta/dt$ is the angular rate of expansion of the retinal image of the sphere. D. Regan reminds us that the astronomer Fred Hoyle used this idea in his 1957 science fiction novel *The Black Cloud*, calculating the time that a dark cloud outside the solar system would strike Earth according to this equation:

$$T = \theta/(d\theta/dt)$$

Here, T is the time until collision and θ is the angle of the object (size) to the observer's retina. (Regan pointed out, though, that such changes could equally likely reflect a growing cloud that was not moving at all.) So, baseball batters and hockey goalies probably estimate arrival times in the same manner with visual cues. However, binocular information (comparing the relative velocities in the two retinas) may be important when the ball or puck gets very close.[7]

Calculation of ball velocity based on changes in retinal image size is particularly advantageous in situations requiring a very quick response, since the estimate of speed can be achieved directly from these retinal changes. That is, we don't need to feed this information through the brain's memory database in order to react.

It should come as no surprise that studies indicate that athletes are more skilled at coincidental timing (figuring out just when to swing the bat as the ball arrives over home plate) than nonathletes are. And skill in baseball hitting and catching has been shown to be directly related to the length of time that a ball in flight can be visually followed, as well as smoothness of eye pursuit movements. Skilled batters are better able to predict where and when the ball will cross the plate than we are. That would seem rather obvious.

In real life, I would never be able to block back one of Andy Roddick's booming serves, but a good number of highly ranked professional players can repeatedly do so. What is not expected, however, is that research studies do not demonstrate particularly large differences in temporomotor coordination abilities between skilled players and nontrained subjects. For instance, in one report about the ability to time the response of swinging a tennis racket with an oncoming light (at a speed of 5 m/s), the accuracy of highly skilled players was only about 15% greater than of that of players with less experience.

A number of studies have been performed to determine just how accurately athletes in different sports can time their motor activity (that is, the variability on multiple attempts).[5] As indicated in the sidebar on this page, these range from 2 to 15 milliseconds, depending on the skill of the athlete and speed of the approaching object. Peter McLeod and his coworkers examined timing accuracy in nonathletic subjects who tried to swing a bat horizontally at a ball dropped down a vertical chute. They found that in 90% of trials, subjects could swing within 10 milliseconds of the approaching ball. They could react within 5 milliseconds in 50% of the trials. McLeod concluded that this information seems rather counterintuitive. Tests of neither coincidental timing nor reaction time appear to be major predictors of sport skill. (One might wonder, however, why the dramatically greater speed of approaching objects in the sport setting has not gained more attention in such comparisons.)

Timing accuracy (variability in multiple trials) in perceptuomotor tasks (standard deviation of coincidental timing, in milliseconds).

Back-leg glance in cricket: + 2 milliseconds

Forehand in table tennis: + 8 milliseconds

Ski jumping (upward thrust at lip of jump): + 10 milliseconds

Catching a ball (closing fingers after ball hits the hand at velocity of 10 m/s): + 15 milliseconds

Response of untrained adults (see preceding text): + 10 milliseconds

Attempt by 9-month-old infants to intercept objects arriving at various speeds: + 50 milliseconds

From various sources.

Anticipation

So, are there other ways by which we can explain the obviously superior skill of athletes in perceptuomotor timing, which, as the following section shows, improves with training? Most likely, the ability to anticipate where and when the ball will arrive, even before or just as the tennis player serves the ball, plays a major role.

A number of investigations in sports, such as baseball, golf, ice hockey, soccer, tennis, and table tennis, have indicated that skilled athletes can better use past experience and visual cues to predict the direction and speed of the ball's flight. For example, it has been reported that expert tennis players were far more proficient at predicting the path of serves by analyzing the server's body position. Skilled players seem to focus more on the area around the server's arm and racket, tracking the ball as it is being tossed, while novices have a variety of visual scanning techniques. As noted previously in this chapter, better baseball players fix their vision on the pitcher's release point to predict direction of the ball. Certainly, factors such as knowledge of an opponent's strengths and weaknesses, the strike count, signals from the coach, and previous patterns of a particular pitcher's delivery would add to predictive ability. As Bruce Abernethy has concluded, "Given the time constraints, especially at the very top level of competition, superior pattern recognition may be an essential precursor to superior anticipation, and in turn, to the ability of expert [tennis] players to give the impression of 'having all the time in the world' to make their return stroke."[8]

Do Athletes Defy the Rules?
Testing the Limits of Perceptual Timing

As we muse over this information, we may have the sense that, considering what neuroscientists tell us about the human limits of perceptual timing skills, the incredible timing abilities of athletes seem almost implausible. Take, for instance, our model of a professional batter attempting to hit a pitched baseball. Considering the tight time constraints during the ball's flight, decision making on the part of the batter would seem limited to the earlier portion—certainly less than the first third—of its trajectory. From what we know about the changes in acceleration and direction of a pitched baseball late in its flight, the batter's tasks of matching the bat's swing with the arrival of the ball and then directing the ball to a vacant sport in the field (which actually occurs around 25% of times at bat) seems beyond belief.

Patricia DeLucia and Edward Cochran, in fact, showed that batters can obtain visual information throughout each portion of the pitched ball's trajectory. They found that blocking the batter's view of any portion of the ball's path caused a reduction in batting accuracy. However, the loss in accuracy was very limited—not more than 20%. And screening the first third of the flight path did not cause a greater decline in batting performance than blocking the middle or the last third.

This information would seem to go against what we know about the limits of visual tracking in humans. It is also contrary to what Adair concluded in the fascinating book *The Physics of Baseball*: "If it weren't psychologically upsetting, the batter could just as well close his eyes after the ball is halfway to the plate, or if it were a night game, management could turn out the lights—the hitter would hit the ball just as well."[3] There has to be some wizardry in these athletic skills that goes beyond an understanding of nerve cell function and organization. (In this category of athletic magic, it has been suggested that baseball batters can actually watch the seams of the ball arriving at 100 mph [160 kmph] to make hitting decisions. They'd have to watch pretty closely. A typical fastball spins at a rate of 1,600 revolutions per minute—about 11 rotations—on its way to the plate.)

What Training Studies Say About Improvement

Getting back to musicians, whether the virtuoso violinist is born or made is open to debate. I'm going to guess that when this is figured out, the answer will be akin to what we currently think about athletes. There are significant genetic influences at two levels: physical capability to perform and the magnitude of the ability to improve with training.

That is, you've got to have the right parents and you've got to practice. There seems to be no question that repeated musical performance—practice—is effective in improving the neuromuscular timing, the speed, and the aesthetic abilities we call musical skills. To get to Carnegie Hall, you do need to practice, practice, practice. And it's not just your mother saying this. It's been reported that violinists who were considered to be excellent performers by age 21 have spent twice as much time in their lives practicing as the average player has (10,000 hours versus 5,000 hours).[9] (But, cries the skeptic, which way does the arrow of causality go here? Couldn't one argue that it might be just as likely that the highly talented violinist, being more motivated and feeling a greater need, would spend more time in the practice room?) Many have concluded that the amount of time devoted to concentrated practice is the single most effective means of acquiring musical expertise. (On the other hand, Mom, one must appreciate genetic limits. I could practice 8 hours daily for years and never be an Andrés Segovia.)

The basic idea, of course, is that in being repeated over and over, the finely timed patterns of muscular expression that go into music performance get *grooved*, or programmed, into the nervous system. That concept has pedagogical implications. For example, piano teachers tell their students to begin a new piece by playing it very slowly—not just because it is easier that way, but also because it prevents errors and engrains the correct notes.

For athletes, the story seems to be the same. There is no question from our common observations that athletes get better with training, that point guards get faster and shoot more accurately and that soccer goalies block more shots as they pass through high school, college, and into the professional ranks. In sports where it counts, all the skills of visuomotor timing enumerated in this chapter (except simple reaction time) also improve with training. (It is important to note, though, that such gains are typically highly task specific. That is, a baseball batter gets better at hitting a pitched ball, but his ability to time a jump for a rebound on the basketball court will remain limited.) The basis for improvement in these sports, then, is largely that of enhancing neuromuscular coordination and timing abilities. It follows, then, that one way to improve such perceptuomotor function—and thereby improve performance—is to simply play and practice a lot.

Considering the critical importance of visuomotor timing in many sports, it has been proposed that specific perceptual training might be useful for athletes. The jury still seems to be out on whether these programs actually work, but many scholars are skeptical. For instance, Abernethy commented that "approaches that might be expected to be of limited value would include generalized training programs (in which the intent is to improve generic visual skills through the use of repetitive training on non-task-specific stimuli), visual search pattern matching, and approaches based on the conscious processing of perceptual information. Generalized visual training programs have been popularized by sports optometrists, but systematic evidence indicating their effectiveness in actually improving sports performance is scarce."[8] That is to say, even in those studies in which perceptual training has been found to improve particular reaction or decision times, there is no indication that such responses can actually be translated into enhanced sport performance in the field. So, whether athletic teams should employ neurophysiologists along with the usual cadre of nutritionists, trainers, and sport psychologists remains to be seen.

Descartes Meets Tim Noakes: Does Self-Determinism Really Exist?

How much do we control our own destiny? Do we truly have free will to choose and alter the events of our lives? Or are we simply players in an unwinding film that is already recorded? You might think it odd that weighty issues that have troubled philosophers for centuries should be raised in this discussion. But bear with me.

The previous sections show that athletic events of extremely short duration—hitting Andy Roddick's first serve—must necessarily occur at an automatic, subconscious level. In contrast, cognitive, conscious decisions can be made for those occurring at least over several seconds. Consider the punt returner who is trying to decide whether to call for a fair catch or not. The punt is high in the air. He judges the time it will take it to descend to earth, recognizes the speed (and combined weight) of the offense's punt coverage team converging on him, dimly knows which yard line he is standing on, and assesses the effectiveness of the wall of blockers on the right side of the field. He actually has time to think about all this and come to a reasonable decision. Or does he?

In a famous set of experiments in the 1980s, Benjamin Libet and his research team raised the surprising (and I dare say, disturbing) idea that actions we normally consider to be set into motion by our own conscious decision making might possibly be already made for us by our subconscious brains. They found that subjects decided to perform a voluntary, spontaneous task (flexing the wrist) 150 to 200 milliseconds before the act. That conscious decision was made, however, 350 to 400 milliseconds after the appearance of electrical potentials on an electroencephalogram that signaled preparation for the action. Thus, "it seems possible that the brain's [unconscious] activities that initiate a willed act begin well before the conscious will to act has been adequately developed."[10]

So, does this mean that we are not really in control of our actions, that they instead are devised by unconscious forces? For many, that would be a disturbing thought. On this point, though, one aspect of these studies seemed to hold out help for believers in free will. In the 100 to 200 milliseconds before the act was performed, there was sufficient time for the conscious self to change, or veto, the act. So, maybe we're in charge after all.

We see this quandary of self-determinism versus the actions of the subconscious brain in other aspects of time perception in athletes. Chapter 1 outlines a similar metaphysical muddle in discussing pacing strategies for long-distance runners. As has been traditionally supposed, does the runner select, from the start, the proper pace that will deliver him to the finish line of a 10K race just before marked fatigue ensues? Does self-determinism rule? (Descartes taught this, albeit admittedly in a different context.)

Or are we just being presumptuous? Does, instead, a central governor in the brain figure this out, keeping the pace safe (avoiding coronary insufficiency, muscle tetany, hyperthermia) through feelings of fatigue, all at an unconscious level? This is the viewpoint of Tim Noakes and his colleagues in South Africa.

I suppose the only presumptuous beings here would be those who claim to know the answers. The issue is intriguing, fundamental,

An Epic Battle of Wills

"There's time distortion when you are in the alpha state—like a hypnotic state. I had no idea that six and half hours had passed." Six and a half hours. Jean Hepner and Vicki Nelson had just set the world's record for the longest continuous professional tennis match. (This was 1984, predating John Isner and Nicolas Mahut in their epic 11-hour battle on the grass at Wimbledon in 2010). And it only went two sets.

The other record set that September day was even more remarkable. For 29 minutes, the two (ranked 172 and 93 in the world, respectively) battled it out for a single point. The 643-point rally ended when Nelson came to net and drove home an overhead smash of Hepner's lob. "Just thinking about it, my stomach is starting to hurt," Hepner later told *New York Times* reporter Dave Seminara. In his article, titled "The Day They Belabored the Point," he relates that Nelson, who eventually won the match, 6-4, 7-6 (11), collapsed with leg cramps, for which she was awarded a time-violation warning by the still-conscious chair umpire.

So, how do you hit straight 322 shots without an error? Said Hepner, "I was just really concentrating."

and not easily amenable to experimental study. One cannot help imagining the creation of entire university departments, international congresses, and journals devoted to a new field of existential philosophy of athletic competition.

Can Athletes Slow Down Time?

We've all heard stories from survivors of serious automobile accidents and similar crisis situations who describe that in the midst of the event, everything just seemed to slow down. The approaching car, the impact, the automobile rolling over all appeared to float in time. "It was just like it was all happening in slow motion." (One might suppose, in fact, that such a suspension of time is necessary if a person's entire life is going to flash in front of his eyes. And, as one of my children once graciously remarked, in my case, that would be a lot of reels.) There is a certain consistency in the nature of these accounts, as Russell Noyes and Roy Kletti found when they collected descriptions of 61 such events. This is, in the end, "a disputed phenomenon for which there is, nevertheless, a wealth of anecdotal evidence."[11]

It's said that athletes can experience similar extensions of time in the midst of intensive competition. Baseball hitters have described a blazing fastball as almost standing still in front them just before contact with the bat. At the Vancouver Winter Olympics, Apolo Ohno explained that in the final lap of a short track skating race, "everything slows down. . . . everything gets quiet." Michael Jordan reportedly stated that as he dribbled by converging opponents, all the action became very slow and deliberate. (From my luxury box, however, any suspension of the time clock was not at all evident.) In his classic book *The Inner Game of Tennis*, Tim Gallwey describes the ball as appearing larger and moving slower when one focuses to return a shot. It is just to this illusion of marked slow motion, this suspension of time, that Jimmy Connors is said to have attributed much of his championship success on the court. In the movies, too, we witness filmmakers using this technique to heighten the dramatic effect of sport action (*Hoosiers*, for example).

Oliver Sacks considered this capability of athletes to slow down time at critical points of competition to be an effect of years of training: "Their neural representation becomes so ingrained in the nervous system as to be almost second nature, no longer in need of conscious effort or decision. One level of brain activity may be working automatically, while another, the conscious level, is fashioning a perception of time, a perception that is elastic and can be compressed or expanded."[11] Others have seen slowing of time in athletic activity as an outcome of intense concentration. Thus, it should be available even to recreational athletes with the right mind-set.

Since these experiences are subjective, it is difficult not only to document such moments of retardation of time but also to study and understand them. Given the frequency with which such time-slowing events have been reported to occur, though, it is reasonable to conclude that they have truth on some level, that they represent some real psychological phenomenon. It would be, too, a reaction to stress that provides value—time to act and avoid accidents, to save people in danger, and, for the athlete, to perform in difficult competitive situations.

In his book *The Labyrinth of Time*, Michael Lockwood points out that another dimension to such reports exists. In addition to the slowing of time, there is a sensation of being "capable of reacting with remarkable alacrity and effectiveness—such as they would normally expect of themselves only if events really were unfolding at the obligingly modest rate that the illusion projects." Such shifts in time perception, he contends, are triggered by events in which "normal powers are in danger of falling short of what circumstance demands of us."[11]

Assuming that moving the athlete's time projector in slow motion is (a) a real phenomenon and is (b) beneficial to sports performance, is it possible to turn it on? As previously noted, Gallwey (and others) have felt that focus and concentration are crucial to altering time perception for improving sports performance. He was talking about tennis and the need to free yourself from thinking too much, from trying too hard, from letting your instinctive abilities play the game. Consciousness is always getting in the way. Concentration in a calm mind is the key. He offered a concrete way of accomplishing this: Focus on the seams of the tennis ball as it crosses over the net toward you. The outcome is that "sometimes the ball even begins to appear bigger or to be moving slower" by the time it reaches you. (I've tried this, and it might work, but my 3.5 rating hasn't budged.) These are "natural results of the concentration of one's conscious energy."[11] From this, some have suggested that meditation and other relaxation practices might aid in altering time perception. (So, this chapter encompasses both existential philosophy and the world of Zen.)[11]

Notes

1. The following is an excellent source of ideas about how our brains perceive time: Gibbon, J., and C. Malapani. 2001. "Neural basis of timing and time perception." In *Encyclopedia of cognitive science*, ed. I. Nadal. Oxford: Oxford Press.

2. Wilson, F.R. 1991. "Music and the neurology of time" *Music Education Journal* 77: 26-30. ———.1988. "Brain mechanisms in highly skilled movements." In *The biology of music making*, ed. F.L. Roehmann and F.R. Wilson, 77-93. St. Louis: MMB Music.

3. Read more about the complexity of hitting a pitched baseball in the following sources: Adair, R.K. 2002. *The physics of baseball*. 3rd ed. New York: Harper Collins. DeLucia, P.R., and E.L. Cochran. 1985. "Perceptual information for batting can be extracted throughout a ball's trajectory." *Perceptual Motor Skills* 61: 143-150. Kindel, S. 1983. "The hardest single act in all of sports." *Forbes* 132: 180-186. Watts, R.G., and A.T. Bahill. 2000. *Keep your eye on the ball. Curveballs, knuckleballs, and fallacies of baseball*. New York: W.H. Freeman and Company.

4. Ted Williams was a perfectionist, and he spent a good deal of time studying and thinking about the pitchers he faced. He also wiped off his bats with alcohol every night to get rid of any resin deposit. He claimed that condensation and dust can add to their weight, and he often took his bats down to the post office and had them weighed. (It was said he could tell the difference himself of a half ounce.) He had 20/10 vision but denied the claim that he could read labels on revolving phonograph records. You can read more about Ted Williams and his batting strategies in his book: Williams, T., and J. Underwood. 1970. *The science of hitting*. New York: Simon and Schuster.

5. Cricket is just as difficult: McLeod, P., and S. Jenkins. 1991. "Timing accuracy and decision time in high-speed ball games." *International Journal of Sport Psychology* 22: 279-285.

6. References for studies of athletes' reaction times: Kida, N.S., S. Oda, and M. Matsumura. 2005. "Intensive baseball practice improves the go-no-go reaction time but not the simple reaction time." *Cognitive Brain Research* 22: 257-264. Lee D.N., D.S. Young, P.E. Reddich, S. Lough, and M.H.T. Clayton. 1983. "Visual timing in hitting an accelerating ball." *Quarterly Journal of Experimental Psychology* 35A: 333-346.

7. If you're thirsting for some hard science and math in regard to tracking oncoming balls, try this article: Regan, D. 1997. "Visual factors in hitting and catching." *Journal of Sports Science* 15: 533-558.

8. Abnernathy, B. 1996. "Training the visual-perceptual skills of athletes. Insights from the study of motor expertise." *American Journal of Sports Medicine* 24: S89-S92.

9. Reference that practice makes perfect: Ericsson, K.A., R.T. Krampe, and C. Tesch-Roma. 1993. "The role of deliberate practice in the acquisition of expert performance." *Psychological Review* 100: 363-406.

10. These ideas can be found in the following book: Libet, B. 2004. *Mind time. The temporal factor in consciousness*. Cambridge, MA: Harvard University Press.

11. For additional perspectives on the feeling of time slowing, see the following sources: Gallwey, W.T. 1974. *The inner game of tennis*. New York: Random

House. Lockwood, M. 2005. *The labyrinth of time*. Oxford: Oxford University Press. Noyes, R., and R. Kletti. 1977. "Depersonalization in response to life-threatening danger." *Comparative Psychology* 18: 375-384. Sacks, O. 2004. "Speed." *The New Yorker*, August 23, 60-69.

TAKE-HOME MESSAGES

1. In many sports (baseball, tennis, hockey, and cricket), the timing of finely tuned perceptuomotor skills taxes the limits of human neurological function.

2. Through training in these sports, athletes translate enhancement of perceptual skills into improved performance.

3. Whether training programs focused on improving basic perceptual skills are useful in enhancing sports performance remains uncertain.

4. Rapid visuomotor timing decisions by athletes are performed automatically, bypassing brain centers of cognitive awareness and decision making. The possibility has been raised that in events of longer duration, supposedly purposeful decisions in sport are actually expressions of predetermined, subconscious strategies that are based on previous playing experience stored in the mind.

CHAPTER 6

Coaches commonly employ programs with little regard for the background and biological makeup of children and with no guiding concepts, such as training principles. Children are not just little adults, but have complex, distinct physiological characteristics that must be taken into account.

Tudor Bompa, 2000

The expert-performance approach has found ample evidence that children and adolescents do not spontaneously engage in the deliberate practice that ultimately leads to maximal performance.

K. Anders Ericsson et al., 2009

GETTING BETTER ALL THE TIME

The Development of Athletic Skill During the Childhood Years— A Conversation With Bob Malina

I've seen the movie *Giant* maybe three times. So when I placed the phone call to Bob Malina down at his home in Texas, I saw the scene in my mind's eye. Professor Malina was probably sipping lemonade out on the veranda of his sprawling ranch home. Before him were the sweeping vistas of the coastal plain, with seas of grass and cattle stretching horizon to horizon. Forests of oil derricks. Maybe Elizabeth Taylor. (No, I was later informed. The cattle ranch belongs to his mother-in-law, not Elizabeth Taylor. Oil wells are things of the past, and the local residents are trying to block a coal-fired power plant on the horizon.)

I had told Bob that I was writing this chapter on the development of athletic talent. About the time between early childhood and the early adulthood, when a training athlete's ability to perform in sports steadily improves, a discrete window of opportunity exists for turning this rise into elite performance. The age of peak performance varies by sport and among individual athletes, yet every event presents a certain time deadline. After this time, even with continued training, performance heads south.

Many question how athletes should be trained within this time constraint. Most particularly, I was wondering about the controversial issue of if, how, and when sport training should be started with young children. Could I talk with him and get his ideas on this?

Bob was gracious enough to agree. This was a stroke of good fortune, for there probably is no one on the planet with greater expertise in the science of developing young athletes. Professor Malina has a double doctorate—one in anthropology (University of Wisconsin), the other in physical education (University of Pennsylvania). He spent much of his career at the University of Texas before moving on to Michigan State. His research has provided the details for how sport performance is related to growth and development in children. He has a teaching legacy, too. An impressive cadre of former students has achieved prominence in the scientific field of pediatric exercise.

Every time I meet up with Bob, I recall participating in a conference in Hong Kong with him a few years back. While touring the city, I made the error of treating Bob and his fellow colleague Colin Boreham to a quick cup of coffee at the Peninsula Club. My gaffe was rapidly disclosed when the check arrived bearing a demand for $35 U.S. Sadly, I could have easily avoided the error if I had noted the fleet of Rolls-Royce vehicles stationed in front of the hotel. (The astute reader will recall, in fact, that this exact scene is portrayed in the James Bond movie *The Man With the Golden Gun*.)

But I digress.

A Pertinent Topic

Rowland: Bob, this whole business of figuring out how to improve physical prowess on the athletic field in the 15 odd years that time permits is really a complicated one, isn't it? Some exercise scientists have spent their whole professional lives trying to sort this out. At a basic level, they've sought to gain insights into just how our motor abilities can be improved. That has importance not only for understanding physiological principles, but also for taking care of people with all sorts of chronic diseases, like those in cardiac and pulmonary rehabilitation programs, and for patients with neuromuscular disorders, such as cerebral palsy.

It's within the world of sports, though, that the importance of success has become so crucial (dare I say exaggerated?) in contemporary society. Here, the question has gained critical importance. There's the father who's just fashioned a tennis ball to swing above the crib of his 6-month-old son, hoping for a head start in his son's future entry into the Australian Open. There's the head of the U.S. Olympic training center who needs to know how he can identify talented swimmers at an early age. The parents of a 10-year-old who just sank five shots in a row from the key in her last game can't decide if they should let her travel with the AAU junior team or if they should enlist her in several different sports. And the director of a youth football league is up to his waist in anxious parents who don't think his practice of matching competitors by age is appropriate.

Malina: It has to be realized that there are no simple answers to how athletic talent can or should be developed—not to mention predicted—within the time constraints of the first part of life. Many factors contribute to sport skill, many factors influence how these can be improved over time, and many factors affect how indicators of athletic performance at an early age might or might not predict later success in the competitive arena.

Rowland: But let's see if we can tease out some of the answers, or at least talk about what researchers think about these things.

Malina: Okay.

Rowland: Because this is such a complex subject, maybe it would be best if we start at the very beginning and then build a story from there. Let's look at figure 6.1.

Malina: I don't see a figure 6.1.

Rowland: You'll see it when the book is published. Trust me on this, Bob.

Malina: Okay.

Rowland: A good starting place is to state that during the growing years, physical performance steadily advances up until late adolescence, on the average, in just about every motor activity you can think of. Running a 50-meter dash, throwing or kicking

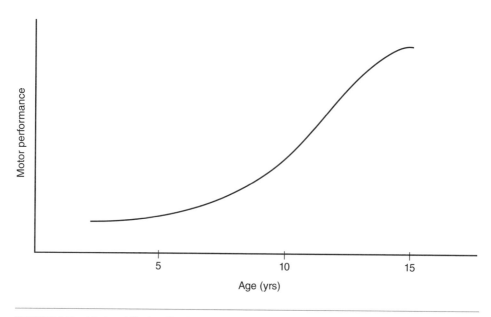

FIGURE 6.1. Motor skills (vertical axis), such as running speed and muscle strength, normally improve with age (horizontal axis) during the course of childhood and adolescence.

a ball, lifting weights. They all improve with age. A 15-year-old boy can run a mile (1.6 km) almost twice as fast as a 6-year-old can. A 14-year-old girl can jump twice as high as she could 10 years earlier. At age 6, the average boy can throw a softball 12 meters, but he can fire it 50 meters at age 15. So, performance in basic athletic skills improves dramatically as children grow, even if they do nothing but sit in front of the television every day after school. That's what we see in figure 6.1. The horizontal axis is age, the vertical axis is performance on a motor task. We recognize this as a basic biological trend on which we can base the rest of our discussion.

Malina: You can see that this is going to be a major challenge for those who study the effects of athletic training on children. They'll have to be able to separate out any effect of programs of skill development and training from those that accompany the normal growth, maturation, and developmental improvements that occur during childhood and adolescence.

Rowland: What factors are most responsible for this natural improvement in motor abilities as children grow?

Malina: This increase in athletic prowess is largely due to increase in body dimensions and neuromuscular maturation. Children get stronger as they grow, largely because their muscles increase in size. They can perform better on aerobic endurance events because their legs are longer (which translates to longer strides) and they have bigger hearts and circulatory systems. And so on. So, the actions of growth hormones and other growth-promoting agents are mainly responsible for these steady improvements in sport abilities with age.

Rowland: Now you have to picture figure 6.2, Bob, which points out the next step: This curve of improving performance abilities during childhood is affected by genetics. If you think back on the second grade, before any training whatsoever, some kids in the class were very fast or very strong, and some weren't. Some of them inherited top-quality performance genes from their parents, others weren't so lucky. In figure 6.2, there are some parallel lines above and below that of our average child, showing that genes that alter the physical and physiological factors that influence performance can affect the curve of motor development.

Malina: I think your readers may be surprised that you can remember back to the second grade, Tom.

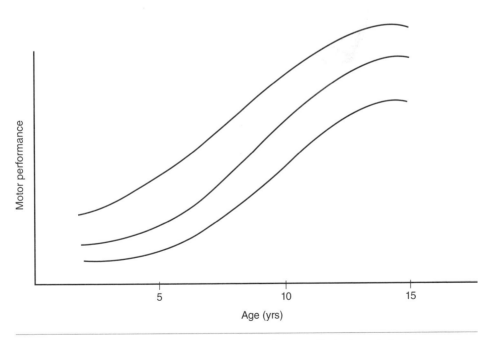

FIGURE 6.2. Levels of motor skill are influenced by genetic factors during the growing years.

Rowland: An unforgettable year. Somewhere around the dawn of electric lighting.

Malina: Now, I can guess that your next step will be what happens when the child reaches puberty.

Rowland: Right. That's when things start getting complicated. During male puberty, surges in testosterone trigger increases in height, muscle bulk, heart size, blood volume, and hemoglobin concentration, all of which improve sport performance. (Girls, on the other hand, gain more body fat, which impedes performance in some sports like gymnastics. But let's stick to just the males for now.) So far, that's clear. The complicating factor is that in any group of youngsters, the pubertal events that trigger all these changes occur at different ages and at different rates. For some youths, performance-enhancing pubertal changes occur early. Others experience them later in adolescence. They also occur at different tempos. Some youths go through the process very quickly in a concentrated manner, while for others, the entire process is drawn out over time. Level of sexual development, with its implications for sport performance, does not follow the youngster's chronological age. That's what figure 6.3 shows.

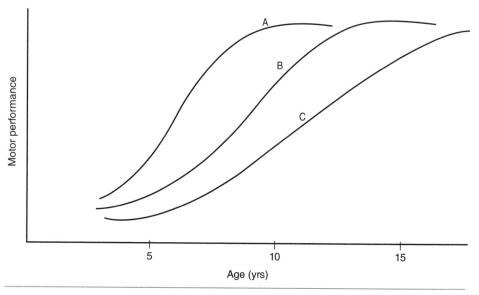

FIGURE 6.3. During puberty, the influence of androgenic hormones (testosterone) in males stimulates growth of musculoskeletal and circulatory systems, which promote exercise performance. The timing and rate of this change can vary markedly by chronological age. A = early maturer, B = average maturer, C = late maturer.

Malina: Think about the implications here. In any group of 12-year-old boys, the early sexual maturers are generally stronger, faster, and more athletically talented. Their hormones have beat the clock, you might say. These boys will be the standout players in youth leagues of football, basketball, baseball, and soccer. It might be supposed that that the late maturers will eventually catch up. By the end of the pubertal period, the effect of differential biological maturation should be reduced, perhaps even erased. The conclusion could be made, then, that trying to predict ultimate basketball talent in college, say, by how a child performs at age 12 might be entirely treacherous, if not impossible. The same applies to other sports. Though early- and late-maturing soccer players differ considerably in size and strength at 11 or 12 years of age, they do not differ that markedly in soccer-specific skills. A key question then becomes how can we protect the small, talented youngster in a given sport?

It's very interesting, then, that the first conclusion—early maturers will be more skillful at younger ages—is true, but maybe the second—that it all evens out in the end—is not. This comes to light when sport success is analyzed by birth date. Since competition is grouped by age category in most youth sports, a child who is born at the first part of the qualifying year can be expected to be bigger—and perhaps more skillful in strength and power activities—than one whose birth date is in the later part of the year. Yet both will be playing at the same level of team competition.

Effect of Birth Date

Malina: Numerous studies have documented this effect.[1] Rosters of participants in youth sports, particularly hockey, are biased toward those with birth dates in the first portion of the year, as compared to the last. The usual explanation is that those who are chronologically older are also more likely to be more biologically mature—stronger, heavier, and taller—offering a competitive advantage. No surprises here. Yet it is intriguing that this same bias for early birth date is seen in highly successful young-adult athletes after puberty as well. Studies of competitors in professional baseball, ice hockey, soccer, and basketball have all indicated a skewing of birthdates toward the quarter of each sport year. Somehow, the early maturers, who are more talented early on, seem to have continued to dominate in their sport. How to explain this? I believe that the size and performance advantages of early maturing boys within their respective age groups attract the attention of coaches and others interested in the search for talent.

Rowland: Before leaving this point, it should be added that in addition to birth date, location of birth also seems to be important. If you want to be a star athlete, grow up in Austin, not New York City or Miller's Corners. Well, that's a bit of hyperbole, but the point is that studies indicate a disproportionate number of professional athletes grow up in cities with populations less than 500,000 but greater than 10,000. Psychosocial environment seems to have some importance in the pathway to sport success. For example, Jean Côté and coworkers reported that about half of the U.S. population lives in cities with more than 500,000 inhabitants, but these cities account for only 13% of National Hockey League players, 29% of professional basketball players, 15% of participants in major league baseball, and 13% of the players in the Professional Golf Association.[2]

Malina: Agreed. Did they provide any explanation for these findings?

Rowland: Well, you can pick your favorite explanation among the many offered: better physical environment of the smaller cities with more unstructured play activities permitting experience in different sports, more local support for sport teams, less competitive milieu, greater chance for early success, and so on.

Malina: So, where did you grow up, Tom?

Rowland: Alma, Michigan.

Malina: That explains everything.

Rowland: Could be. So, remember, we have been talking here about the steady, normal improvements in motor performance that occur as children grow. No training, just normal development, governed by growth-promoting hormones and affected by genetic endowment and level of sexual development.

Malina: We should add a third component, behavioral development, to this normal progression, too. This is a cultural concept. In their social milieu, children develop cognitively, socially, emotionally, and morally—they are learning to behave within the constructs of our society. This also applies to motor development and sports, specifically societal expectations and rewards associated with proficiency or lack of proficiency. The demands of sports may influence, or even sometimes conflict, with this normal behavioral development.

All three of these trends—physical growth, biological maturation, and behavioral development—are in a state of constant change and interaction during childhood and adolescence, and the rates of change and interactions vary greatly from one child to the next. So when thinking about the effects of sport training on children, we must appreciate that adult-organized programs are superimposed on a constantly changing base.

Rowland: Let's turn now to the effect of athletic training on the natural progression of events. To what extent can athletic training accelerate the normal improvements in physical performance of children and adolescents as they grow (that is, beyond the stimuli provided by Mother Nature)? And, as a corollary, can a child's ultimate development into a performing athlete be enhanced by early sport training?

Just to be clear, by *training*, we mean a program of systematic instruction and practice of certain frequency, intensity, and duration. That improvement in sport skill should be achieved through training is based on the precept that regular exercise stresses body tissues, which, in response, compensate by improving function. That function is then translated into greater performance outcomes. Also, in sports involving complex neuromuscular skill, such as tennis, there is the concept that repeated practice grooves neuromuscular connections, providing a kind of muscle memory.

Malina: It should be readily apparent that when thinking about the applicability of these principles to youth, a number of considerations are important. For instance, are the children at a proper stage of readiness or preparedness to respond to such stimuli in terms of their personal stages of growth and development? Are there critical periods when children are optimally sensitive to improvements associated with instruction and practice (in the case of sport skills) and physical training (regarding biological dimensions and functions)? How do differences in coaching strategies and instructional techniques at different ages make a difference? Our understanding of these issues is very limited.

Peak Performance Ages

At what age should highly trained athletes be expected to reach their peak performance? Obviously, it depends on the sport, and many exceptions to the rule exist. But researchers have committed serious effort trying to pinpoint these average ages. As you thumb through the literature, here's what you'll find:

Baseball players tend to reach their peak pitching and hitting capabilities at 28 or 29 years of age. In tennis, top performance is typically reached at age 24, in golf at 31. In track-and-field events like the shot put, high jump, and pole vault, the peak is usually in the mid 20s. Figure skaters, early 20s. As a general statement, females tend to peak earlier than their male counterparts. There has been a recent trend—tennis is a good example—for greater expertise in younger competitors.

Gymnastics has an interesting story. Many years ago, champions in women's gymnastics were typically in their 20s, and some were much older. In the 1956 Olympics, the individual gold medal went to Hungarian gymnast Agnes Keleti, who was 35 years old. As time went on, the average age of female Olympic gymnasts fell, and medal winners in their mid and late teens were common. As the difficulty in gymnastics increased, so did the intensity of training. In response to concerns of exploitation as well as physical and psychological injury, a rule was instituted in 1976 that competitors had to have reached their 14th birthday. The minimum age for competition in senior-level events has since been raised to 16 years.

In 1994, before the latest age restriction, the average age of international gymnasts was 16.5 years. In 2005, after the new limit, it was 18.1 years. Not all have been in favor of the new minimum age. For gymnastics success, girls need to be favored by small stature, light weight, low body fat, flexibility, and what is called a good strength-to-weight ratio. All of these features can be unfavorably altered at puberty, when the body's center of gravity also changes. Peak performance, at least from a physical standpoint, might occur not long after—if not before—the age of 16 years. Male gymnasts, on the other hand, have a later development of strength-to-weight ratio that is optimal in their early 20s.

One of the most intriguing observations lies in the realm of peak performance in running events. Although some discrepancies among different reports exist, here are the average reported ages by gender:

Event	Men (years)	Women (years)
100 meters	22	21
5,000 meters	25	21
10,000 meters	27	25
Marathon	29	29

Notice any trends here? Again, the women seem to peak earlier than the men. But you'll also see that the longer the race, the older the peak performers. (Those readers approaching the later decades of life can do some arithmetic to figure out at which distance they should now peak out.)

Rowland: Let's begin by considering some examples of physiological fitness. Like muscle strength. It wasn't that long ago that people felt that it was impossible, and maybe even dangerous, for children to try to improve their muscle strength with resistance training, like lifting weights, before puberty. It was thought that you had to have circulating testosterone to do this. But now we know this is false. A good number of studies have documented that children, both boys and girls, gain strength in properly designed programs, just as adults do. So, we should expect that weight training would help children improve performance in sporting events where strength is an issue, most directly in, say, wrestling or powerlifting, but also in football, swimming, and even baseball. The studies haven't been done yet to really prove this, but it makes sense.

Aerobic endurance performance, like distance running, is associated with $\dot{V}O_2$max, the highest amount of oxygen utilized by the body in an exercise test on a cycle or treadmill. With a period of aerobic endurance training, children typically show a rise in $\dot{V}O_2$max, on the average about 5 to 6%. Since that number is less than what is observed in adults (15-20%), some have suggested that this implies that prepubescent children might be less trainable than adults in aerobic endurance sports. But it is not clear if the dampened response of $\dot{V}O_2$max to training in children can be translated into a similarly limited increase in aerobic endurance performance itself. That's because performance on, say, a 5K road race is dependent not only on $\dot{V}O_2$max but also on factors like economy of running energy.

Limited Insights

Malina: Youth athletic programs place a major emphasis on improving motor skills that are more specific to sports, such as throwing, jumping, and ball kicking. Given this focus, it is rather surprising that a very limited amount of research exists on the trainability of such abilities in children. Equally lacking are data to indicate whether particular instructional techniques are more effective than others. And we know little about the influence of variables such as environmental constraints, peer influence, and parent modeling. But from the few investigations that have been done, it does seem that instruction and practice on early acquisition of motor skills is beneficial in improving motor performances in early childhood years (ages 3 to 7).[3]

Even less scientific data exist on the effect of specific instruction and training on gains in sport skills at later and higher levels of competition. It is taken for granted, even by the casual observer, that sport-specific skills generally improve during the course of a season. But, again, the available studies generally support trainability in older children of capabilities in activities, such as baseball pitching, basketball shooting, and soccer skills. Certainly the skill development that appears to occur in the setting of dedicated intensive sport schools involving tennis, skating, and gymnastics would support the meager scientific evidence that youths can respond with significant improvements in performance following appropriate training regimens.

An important area that has lacked previous attention here is the environment of instruction, practice, and coaching in highly specialized programs in all sports. Moreover, I doubt that high-level coaches want their programs systematically studied! If you follow media reports, you'll see that there is much to be desired.

Rowland: So, to sum this up, it does appear that children and adolescents can, in fact, respond with improvements in athletic performance in response to adult-organized training programs. It is reasonable to conclude that the effectiveness of such training depends on the physical and cognitive readiness of the individual child, and that youth training programs need to be designed with this in mind.

But a good many questions remain. If your goal is to produce a high-performance athlete, when in the course of childhood should intensive training be instituted? How can the child who has the capacity for such development be identified? What about the concerns regarding the ethical aspects of early, intense sport training in children? That is, maybe we can train children, but should we? Bob, I hope you have the answers to all these questions.

Malina: Right. And I would add another aspect to your summary—that distinct individual differences exist in responsiveness to instruction, practice, and training programs.

To start with, we can talk all day about these issues, but, in fact, the reality is that the rush to train child athletes continues unabated. We only need to consider parents awakening at 5:00 a.m. to drive their 7-year-old to the hockey rink, the national traveling teams for 10-year-old basketball players, the private coaches and training programs focused on developing child talent, parents holding their children back a year in school to gain an athletic advantage. As Dan Gould has put it, whether we like it or not, we are witnessing the "professionalism of child sports." You can also add the influence of the sporting goods industry to the mix.

Rowland: And whether we are witnessing parents' laudable desires to have their children enjoy themselves and fulfill their physical abilities or, beyond certain limits, children being placed in highly intensive sport training to satisfy the vicarious needs of parents and coaches (in fact violating child labor laws and constituting child abuse) is open to acrimonious debate. So, as we discuss the scientific merits (or lack thereof) of training children, we need to keep in mind the strong cultural and societal forces and sharp controversies that exist on these matters beyond the simply scientific.

Malina: Let's pretend for a moment that we have the luxury of avoiding such conflicts, and dispassionately examine some ideas about what might be the wisest approach, from a scientific standpoint, to developing young talent. There are, in fact, two major camps on this issue. One holds that a certain amount of practice and training is obligatory for talent development. This must be accomplished in a finite amount of time. Consequently, early sport specialization in the growing years is requisite for high-level play, particularly in sports in which peak performance occurs early, like the teen years for gymnastics. The other camp argues that basic steps of developing athletic skill during childhood must occur in stages that incorporate early generalized exposure to different physical activities. This concentration in a particular sport should not occur until later childhood, early adolescence, or perhaps later, depending on the sport. These people argue, too, that "too much, too soon" results in burnout and injuries that will inhibit long-standing participation in sports, rather than encourage it.

Power of Practice

Rowland: Let me talk about the first point of view and then get your opinion. Let's suppose I'm, say, 16 years old, and in the excitement of watching the summer Olympic Games on television, I'm struck with the idea of training hard to become a medal winner in the 5,000-meter run. So, I start a training regimen of regular running, increasing my distance. What will happen to my 5K race times? At the start, I will find rather dramatic improvement from race to race, but as time goes on, that rise in performance will slow. After a few months, I will probably see little change over time, even though I'm still training. And, guess what? My 5K time for that plateau will not be anywhere near what I saw at the Olympic event.

This is the pattern of the typical power law of practice. By the traditional explanation, I have reached my genetic limit for distance running performance. By hereditary constraints, I can never match those Ethiopian runners taking the medals at the 5,000-meter event. I've reached the upper limits of my inherited capabilities and can't surpass them, even with training.

K. Anders Ericsson and his colleagues at Florida State University, among others, have challenged this premise. They would tell me I reached my limit, not because I hit a genetic-determined ceiling, but rather because I failed to employ proper training techniques. They argue that "distinctive characteristics of exceptional performers are results of adaptations to extended and intense practice activities that selectively activate dormant genes that are contained with all healthy individuals' DNA."[4] Those potentiating training techniques are labeled *deliberate practice*, meaning highly focused coach-guided sessions that solely concentrate on improving certain aspects of performance. Simply repeatedly performing the activity, the way I did with my daily runs, will not get me by the plateau. But, with sustained deliberate practice, high levels of performance can be attained.[4]

How long does this take? Ericsson and his coworkers developed their ideas from their studies of musicians—pianists and violinists—showing that performers at the highest level exhibited more deliberate practice patterns. These elite players started training at an earlier age than less-talented performers. A retrospective analysis indicated that these top musicians had accumulated a greater number of practice hours—approximately 10,000 by the time they reached 20 years of age.

Previous studies of chess players suggest that it takes about 10 years to develop the highest levels of grand master expertise. That number was consistent with what Ericsson and colleagues saw with the musicians. The 10-year rule (minimum for this threshold) for achieving elite expertise seems to hold up for athletes, too. People who have examined the courses of development of champion swimmers, distance runners, and tennis players have observed the same thing—elite performance requires at least 10 years of deliberate practice. Researchers have estimated the number of training hours for elite athletes that might be involved over this time span, and it also comes out to somewhere around 10,000. So, we have the popular notion that 10 years and 10,000 hours of practice—the right kind of practice—are necessary to make you a champion athlete.

As the last chapter notes, the weakness of this numerical reasoning is that it is based on a retrospective analysis. Nothing in this information tells us about causality. It could be that naturally highly talented performers are motivated, or have greater opportunities, to practice more.

Anyway, if you believe all this, it is apparent that commitment to sport specialization and intensive training would need to begin early in childhood. Athletes in most sports should be at high levels of performance at least by the time they reach their 20s (and in some cases, like gymnastics, tennis, and figure skating, much earlier). So, a little arithmetic tells us that if would-be champions have to get in all those years and hours, they should be in the gym regularly, with structured coaching, early in their elementary school years.

That parents should believe in this idea is fueled, of course, by the stories we all know of some of the world's very greatest athletes—Andre Agassi, Tiger Woods—whose parents had them training regularly from the time they were toddlers. (I understand that Tiger once beat the comedian Bob Hope in a putting contest on a TV show when he was only 3 years old.) What is ignored here, obviously, is the denominator in such stories. How many 4-year-olds who took daily private tennis lessons at the local club never achieved success?

Perhaps it should be pointed out here that the reader should not confuse the train-them-early approach to sport success with attempts to identify child sport prodigies (we'll be discussing this more a bit later on). When those researchers looked at the course of development of eventual star athletes, they generally found that these elite competitors were not exceptionally gifted early on. They didn't make accelerated improvements in performance with training, either. Their success was gradual. Instead, it seemed related to starting early, gaining access to superior training opportunities, and having the advantage of talented coaches and supportive parents and siblings.

Does Success Breed Success?

Malina: I wonder if the impact of early sport success is not underrated in these kinds of analyses. Children who find themselves doing well when first getting into a particular sport get a lot of ego-fulfilling feedback and, often, the indulgence (wanted or not) of coaches and other adults. Children who start out playing poorly are not motivated to continue and are often eliminated from the sport system—either voluntarily (dropping out) or involuntarily (being cut from the team). Children, like adults, do what they're good at and what they enjoy doing.

Rowland: So, Bob, I have lots of questions for you. What do think of these rules of 10 and early sport specialization in children? Let me really pin you down on this: The father of a 3-year-old who lives next door is determined that she be an Olympic gymnast. He asks you if it's too early to get her into a training program at the local sport club. What do you tell him?

Malina: Tom, I would first ask the father to think about the following questions: Is this for his child or for himself? How does he evaluate the adults who run the program? If it is a developmental gymnastics program that is child-centered and emphasizes basic movement skills, I would have no trouble recommending that he enroll his child. However, he should be sensitive to his daughter's response to the program. Is she really enjoying it? (Young children will not often let on directly, since they want to keep their parents happy. She will, however, tell you indirectly with behavior, comments, and play activities with toys at home.) Try to find out if she really wants to do this. Unfortunately most parents do not listen to their children, talking at them rather than with them.

When I talk to parents about early initiation of sport training during the preschool years, I raise issues (actually red flags) related to the careers of Michael Jackson, Tiger Woods, and other elite individuals who attained success at a relatively young age. I am convinced that preoccupation with a single activity beginning at a very early age, attainment of success at a young age, preferential treatment and indulgence by adults, and the entertainment or sport systems, all influence and perhaps lead to the arrest of other dimensions of normal behavioral development. It is likely that athletes who became successful and specialized at young ages have missed out on many valuable experiences in the normal process of growing up.

To make a long story short, I would encourage the father not to enroll his child in a program aimed at sport specialization at an early age. Childhood should be a smorgasbord of experiences—group and solitary play, social interactions, school, and so on—from which children can learn the broad range of behaviors expected of society.

Rowland: Another school of thought holds that this emphasis on early sport specialization by young children is misguided and may even be detrimental to their future athletic success. The argument is that, yes, elite athletes often have started sport involvement at an early age. Most typically, though, they participated in a variety of activities, not just one, and specialized intensive training in a particular sport did not occur until later on. This pattern of delayed specialization, its advocates contend, provides for better overall development of fitness and motor skills, preventing early athlete burnout and injuries.[5]

In sports like figure skating and gymnastics, in which performance must peak in the teen years, early specialization would seem to be required. But for most other sports, this isn't true. Research bears witness to participants in tennis, field hockey, and soccer who accelerate their training to reach elite levels during the teen years. Competitors who turn out to be expert baseball, rowing, and basketball players have usually involved themselves in a number of different sports early on.

The advantages of this early diversification are supported by certain developmental constructs that cite the value of generalized (rather than specific) motor skills, of playlike participation, and physiological cross-training between activities. As the argument goes, it provides time for the development of intrinsic motivation and other psychological skills important for high-level training (self-confidence, ability to concentrate, capacity for strategizing, and so on).

This approach, its proponents contend, avoids certain risks associated with early sport specialization during childhood. These include impaired psychosocial development from the social isolation that occurs with early training, overuse injuries, and rates of burning out or dropping out.

Tudor Bompa, the famous sport coach who developed young athletes in Romania behind the Iron Curtain in the 1960s, has been one of the strongest advocates for multilateral sport involvement for children at young ages. His experience in the Soviet Union at that time shows the following:

- Most young athletes had a diversified early involvement in sports
- Specialized programs were commonly withheld until 15 to 17 years of age
- Peak performances were achieved 5 to 8 years after specialized training

The children who began sport specialization at an early age demonstrated peak performances at a junior age level. However, these performances were not duplicated when they reached maturity (18 years). Many, in fact, dropped out of sports. Those who had a diversified early sport experience had a slower rate of improvement in performance, peaking at a later age, but demonstrated a high level of persistence and fewer injuries.[6]

Bompa comments, "Specificity training results in faster adaptation, leading to faster increments of performance. But that does not mean that coaches and athletes have to follow it from an early age to physical maturation. This is the narrow approach applied to children's sports, in which the only scope of training is achieving quick results, irrespective of what may happen in the future of the young athlete. It's important for young children to develop a variety of fundamental skills to help them become good general athletes before they start training in a specific sport."

Malina: I agree with Tudor Bompa on multilateral training and the importance of learning a variety of basic skills. But in the former Eastern European sport systems, the multilateral training was essentially under adult supervision at all times. The youth trained within specific sport programs. What is lacking in this approach is time for the youngster to be a child or adolescent, which means participation in informal street games.

Unstructured sport activities are by definition uncharacterized by explicit teaching and adult supervision. They involve much trial and error, experimentation, and unstructured repetition, or practice. It is postulated that skills learned under informal conditions are influenced less by fatigue and stress. Street sports and other unstructured activities obviously vary with the number of youths available and generally change with the season, exposing them to different skills and rules. Such activities in all likelihood involve the learning of sport skills without awareness or explicit knowledge of them. The same can probably be said for social interactions and development.

Rowland: I like Jean Côté's take on this issue. He and his colleagues have emphasized that in the optimal approach to early training, sport skills are learned that are appropriate to the child's stage of growth and development. They believe that the essence of deliberate practice, with its hours of focused work, delayed gratification, and need for self-control, is not yet in the grasp of most preadolescent athletes. "By the time athletes reach adolescence," they say, "they will have acquired fundamental movement skills though deliberate play and will have developed mature cognitive skills. At this point, an appropriate shift in training would include more complex kinds of learning and deliberate practice activities."[7] So, they're saying that, yes, sustained deliberate practice is important, but, no, young children are not yet developmentally ready for this type of commitment.

So, what we've been discussing here is talent development, how athletic potential can best be realized through training, all within a limited time span. You can see that no one's quite sure. If I might be so bold as to try to summarize: It seems the conflict lies between constraints of time available for deliberate practice and the developmental readiness of the young child. If all children were the same in such developmental progress—physically, psychologically, socially—it would all be at least a bit easier. But, no.

Malina: I, too, agree with the approach of Jean Côté, but the issue goes beyond the relatively simple dichotomy of time constraints for deliberate practice and developmental readiness. This viewpoint overlooks the normal demands of growth, maturation, and development—that is, the normal demands of growing up. I personally believe it is abnormal for a child to willingly and knowingly devote several hours per day to the specific repetitive practice of a sport or musical instrument. If it truly was the child's choice—and not that of an overinvolved parent—I might modify my view. But it seems to me that children have too much else to do, engaging in play that is free, imaginative, and social.

Early Identification of Talent

Rowland: Now that we've got that all nailed down, let's move on and talk a bit about early talent identification. How can we initially identify the special child who is ultimately destined for athletic stardom, the one who deserves coaching and developmental training programs? Certainly it would be hard to overstate the importance of this issue to those whose careers—reflecting the success of teams, their universities, cities, and nations—are focused on producing elite athletic talent.

Malina: There are a variety of approaches to early talent identification, but the structured approach that was characteristic of Eastern European countries and, more recently, of China has received the most attention. In this method, which is sometimes labeled the *scientific approach,* young children are identified through screening at an early age, usually on the basis of general motor proficiency (motor development) and physical characteristics. Those doing the screening have a general idea of the physical characteristics associated with specific sports. Those who are so identified are then directed into specific programs for more specialized evaluation. Ages at screening, it should be noted, vary with the sport.

Take diving, for example. In addition to height, weight, and physique, strength, speed, power, muscular endurance, and flexibility are basic components of fitness required for the sport. You could also add spatial orientation, balance control, rhythmic sensitivity, and acoustic and optical reactions as being important perceptuomotor characteristics of a talented diver. Youths who score well on tests for these characteristics may be selected for diving development programs.

The same may be done for team sports. Soccer, for example, requires speed, power, agility, and aerobic endurance, in addition to control of the feet and body, accuracy in shooting and passing, and perceptuocognitive skills. Youths who score well on a battery of tests of these abilities would likely be identified for soccer development programs.

This is a classic approach that's been used for many sports, especially in the selection programs in Eastern European countries. It is being used now in some sports in Australia and China. On the surface, at least, it seems to have shown success. However, you only hear about the successes, and you don't know the denominator in the equation to calculate success. The basis of this approach, of course, lies in the assumption that early sport-related traits are predictive of those later on. The problem is, as noted above, there is no way such a supposition can be expected.

Here's a word of caution about the sport selection programs in Eastern Europe. Tudor Bompa has highlighted the success of the talent identification programs in the former German Democratic

Republic (GDR) and Bulgaria, in which 80% of the medalists came from this type of program. The success of the GDR athletes was especially evident in swimming, particularly for females. However, 12 years later, attention was brought to records of hormonal doping of these competitors. One can thus ask, were the athletes selected or were they experimental subjects?

Rowland: So, I would guess that with this approach, there would be a large number of dropouts, or failures. At the same time, some athletes who matured later but had the potential for success would be missed altogether.

Malina: You are correct. In the structured systems, you only hear about the successes, and you do not know the denominator for the equation to calculate success. Nonetheless, sport governing bodies have made major investments in the method. It's not difficult to see that a good number of other problems exist in taking this route to identify early signs of athletic talent. Clearly, the physical and physiological measures that are being used don't really get at all the factors that go into talent. Sometimes athletes can be very successful by compensating in one area for another in which they aren't so strong. Yet, they'd flunk the testing battery based on that weakness. And psychological qualities, which are so critical for sport success, are generally totally ignored. Of relevance for team sports, too, is game intelligence. A youngster may have the requisite physical and skill characteristics, but may not be able to see the field in soccer, anticipate a pass, move to a space, and so on. Overall, the predictive value of early testing batteries has to be very low. Obviously, the older the child when such testing is undertaken, the better the results in terms of predictability.

Rowland: Attempts at early identification of sport talent are extraordinarily complex. We've got all these determinant variables that are changing as the child grows. Between different youngsters, the rate of change varies and the outcome level of skill and its timing seems quite unpredictable. It's interesting that people who have a keen interest in analyzing multilayered, multifaceted problems like this—they're called dynamic system theorists— have actually given a good deal of thought to the issue of early talent identification. They've likened the nonlinear dynamics of talent development to chaos theory, in which very small perturbations in initial conditions can create major amplifying effects. That makes outcome prediction essentially impossible (long-term weather forecasting being the model).

Writing in the journal *Nonlinear Dynamics, Psychology, and Life Sciences*, Angela Abbott and her coworkers in Edinburgh have commented that "while this message suggests a rather bleak outlook for those wishing to predict future characteristics or behaviors of an athlete (that accurate long-term predictions are impossible), an important distinction must be made. Human performers possess a critical quality (to a greater extent than other chaotic systems) in their ability to display intentional, goal-directed behavior. Humans can be seen as deterministic organisms. . . . and individuals with sufficient drive and determination are more likely to overcome barriers and physical shortcomings in order to be successful in the future than those who do not possess such qualities."[8]

Malina: If I understand the dynamic systems approach to motor development and skill acquisition correctly, the process involves the interactions of three constraints: the child or performer, the environments (natural, manmade, and social), and the specific movement task. These all change and interact as the child grows. Specific instruction and practice represent a manipulation of only one component of the environment. This element is undoubtedly important in skill development, but it cannot be treated in isolation from other components of the environment and, of course, from the child himself.

An Alternative Approach

Rowland: The other major approach is more informal, promoting mass participation in a sport by young children and then letting those with the most talent identify themselves as they grow older. This method has been called weeding out, letting the cream rise to the top, or the last man standing.

Malina: This is the usual early-selection process in the United States and westernized countries (one thinks particularly of swimming, soccer, and baseball) in which there is a large pool of young athletes. The focus is more on demonstrated performance rather than on physical characteristics and specific test skills that characterize the more structured approach.

American football and basketball are somewhat in between, given the emphasis on size as a selective factor. So, the seemingly informal programs may be more formal than meets the eye. Youngsters participating in these sports are under constant observation and scrutiny, especially by other coaches, interested adults, school and club administrators, potential agents, and athletic management programs. These adults are looking for talent, which from their perspective is essentially a commodity to be marketed. Once athletically gifted children are noted, these adults may try to enroll them in select programs or on a travel team. In some cases, they may encourage parents to enroll their children in a specific middle or high school. What I am trying to say here is that the seemingly informal programs have a very formal dimension when it comes to youths who have demonstrated their talent in local competitions.

Tudor Bompa has correctly noted that there is an element of chance here—the development of a child's athletic potential would rest on the chance that he chose to participate early on in a sport for which he had ultimate talent. How many extraordinary lugers are there in the United States who never participated in the sport? How many Michael Jordans are hidden in the Inuit population?

Rowland: Which approach do you think is best?

Malina: There's no simple answer to this question. There are too many variables involved in this process of talent identification and development, most of which are beyond the control of coaches, the sport system, and even the athletes themselves. To start with, how would we even define *success*? Many would look at the medal count in the Olympic Games. But what we're seeing there is only the numerator of our question—those who are successful. We usually don't have information regarding the denominator, or the total number of athletes identified and selected.

What is the chance of success from participation in youth sport at the elite level? It's not very high! Here's an example. In Russia in the 1990s, 2 million youths 6 to 15 years old were said to be participating in sports, which was around 10% of that age group. Of these, 35,000 enlisted in specific sport-training schools. This number was narrowed down to 2,700 who competed on national teams. Of these, 49 were considered to be competing at elite levels. That turns out to be 0.14% of the athletes who were enrolled in intensive sport training. People have done this kind of analysis and found similar success rates for the Chinese at the Beijing Olympics in 2009, elite sport schools in Germany, and the probability that a high-school athlete in the United States will move into the professional ranks. The nature of sport is selective and exclusive!

Tom, I don't think we can allow ourselves to close this topic without offering a summary of personal opinion.

Rowland: Let's do it. We're probably safe. Most readers have probably dropped out a few pages back, anyway.

Malina: Early specialization in a year-round sport has become increasingly common for talented young children. Many factors are responsible for this trend, including pressure from parents, the desire for scholarships or professional contracts, the goals of the sporting goods and services industry, and even ourselves, the sport scientists. The early careers of most high-level athletes, on the other hand, are marked by experiences in a variety of sports before specialization. The risks of doing too much, too soon are great—social isolation and manipulation, burnout, and overuse injuries. It's important for us to keep youth sport in perspective. Young athletes are children and adolescents who have the needs of children and adolescents.

Notes

1. A review of the age effect on youth sports can be found in the following article: Musch, J., and S. Grondin. 2001. "Unequal competition as an impediment to personal development: A review of the relative age effect in sport." *Developmental Review* 21:147-167.

2. Côté, J., D.J. MacDonald, J. Baker, and B. Abernethy. 2006. "When 'where' is more important than 'when': Birthplace and birth date effects on the achievement of sporting expertise." *Journal of Sports Sciences* 2: 1065-1073.

3. For a review of studies examining the acquisition of motor skills in youth through sports training, see the following article: Malina, R.M. 2008. "Skill acquisition in childhood and adolescence." In *The Young Athlete*, ed. H. Hebestreit and O. Bar-Or, 96-111. Malden, MA: Blackwell Publishing.

4. Anders Ericsson, K., K. Nandagopal, and R.W. Roring. 2009. "Toward a science of exceptional achievement." *Annals of New York Academy of Sciences* 1172:199-217. Ericsson, K.A., R.T. Krampe, and C. Tesch-Romer. 1993. "The role of deliberate practice in the acquisition of expert performance," *Psychological Review* 100: 363-406.

5. This article gives a nice outline of the early specialization versus early diversification debate: Baker, Joseph. 2003. "Early specialization in youth sport: A requirement for adult expertise?" *High Ability Studies*, 14: 85-94.

6. Bompa, Tudor. 2000. *Total training for young champions*. Champaign, IL: Human Kinetics.

7. For an argument against early sport specialization, read the following: Côté, Jean, Joseph Baker, and Bruce Abernethy. 2003. "From play to practice: A developmental framework for the acquisition of expertise in team sports." In *Expert Performance in Sports*, ed. J.L. Starkes and K. Anders Ericsson, 89-114. Champaign, IL: Human Kinetics.

8. Read about theoretical models of sport talent identification in the following articles: Abbott, A., C. Button, G.J. Pepping, and D. Collins. 2005. "Unnatural selection: Talent identification and development in sport." *Nonlinear Dynamics Psychology and Life Sciences* 9: 61-88. Vaeyens, R., M. Lenoir, A.M. Williams, and R.M. Philippaerts. 2008. "Talent identification and development programmes in sport." *Sports Medicine* 38: 703-714.

TAKE-HOME MESSAGES

1. Athletic performance reaches a peak during the first portion of life despite continued training. The age at that zenith varies by sport, but all competitors have a certain limited time for optimizing success.

2. Most of the improvements in athletic performance with training occur during the growing years of childhood and adolescence. During this period, motor abilities normally improve due to physical growth and sexual development, though the rate of such gains varies considerably from child to child.

3. Limited data suggest that children can respond with improvements in fundamental and sport-specific motor skills with appropriate sport training.

4. Variations in timing (when) and tempo (how rapidly or slowly) of biological development that are associated with increases in size and strength (males) and body fat content (females) at the time of puberty can affect prediction of future sport success.

5. Two schools of thought dominate talent development: early specialization necessitated by a limited time for skill development (particularly in sports like gymnastics, in which performance peak is early) and early multilateral involvement in sports with later specialization to allow overall fitness gains and to lessen risk of dropout and injuries.

6. Early identification of sport talent is considered important by adults involved in sports but is, in fact, difficult to achieve. The two most common approaches are (a) use of sport-specific physical and physiological profiles and (b) identification of superior performers out of mass participation. Shades of variation exist between the two extremes. The relative success of these two strategies is difficult to ascertain. There are simply too many intervening factors.

CHAPTER 7

Passing through the awkward age, followed by the age of consent, training athletes continue to improve. But once they have achieved the age of discretion, they share with the nonathlete a steady deterioration in physiological function and motor performance. It's all in the process of growing old, the ticking of the ultimate biological clock. Can physical training forestall this decline? This chapter looks at the evidence.

OVER THE HILL
Aging and Sport Performance

Entropy rules. The degree of disorder of a system—organic or inorganic—increases with time. Organization becomes disorganization. In the end, everything runs down. From the jar of mayonnaise on the second shelf, to the 1968 Buick, to the stars of the most distant galaxies. They all disintegrate with the passage of the days, years, or centuries. Indeed, the existence of things is bracketed, is defined, by time. After the hands of the clock have advanced just so far, the mayonnaise is no longer mayonnaise, the Buick is no longer an automobile, the giant red star is no longer a luminary body. It is obvious, then, that time, existence, and entropy are all intimately linked.

Humans run down, too. Our presence on earth as ourselves is dictated by the inexorable course of the years, which, at least physically, will define a lifetime. Like T.S. Eliot's women, we "come and go, talking of Michelangelo." Or, for those preferring the sports vernacular, at the moment of your conception, the shot clock starts up. You've got about 80 years to get a shot off before the buzzer sounds.

But not all is gloom and doom. There are, without doubt, certain advantages to be gained in the aging process (although the list is disappointingly short). Like acquiring wisdom. And lower prices at the movies. Cheaper lift tickets. No more 2:00 a.m. feedings. The time could even be ripe for mature romance. In Gilbert and Sullivan's *The Mikado*, Ko-Ko proposes marriage (albeit reluctantly) to the aged spinster Katisha, singing the following:

Are you old enough to marry, do you think?
Won't you wait until you're 80 in the shade?
There's a fascination frantic
In a ruin that's romantic;
Do you think you are sufficiently decayed?

Athletes, of course, hear the same clock ticking. After a heady couple of decades of steady improvement, personal bests, promises of athletic stardom, and hopes for Olympic gold, it all inevitably starts to deteriorate. Passes fall short, 10K times drift upward, doubles replace singles, knee braces become standard apparel. There is, in fact, probably no area of human endeavor in which biological deterioration with increasing age is so clearly and disappointingly obvious than to those who are trying to push back barriers of motor performance.

So, it is fitting that this book concludes by considering the grandest clock of all, the one that marks off our moments of existence, and just how it influences athletic performance. This chapter discusses what we know about why performance universally declines as we get older and, importantly, if and how such deterioration might be avoided, or at least slowed. As the human life span has increased, this topic has captured an extraordinary degree of both lay and scientific attention. We will thus be limited to but a brief survey of the subject in these few pages. This chapter provides references to more comprehensive works as we move along.

Categories of Aging

Before launching into our topic, the discerning reader should be aware of certain important concepts and cautions. To start with, it should be recognized that two kinds of aging exist. *Primary aging* is an intrinsic process of all human tissues, independent of disease and environmental factors, in which progressive deterioration of cellular integrity and function over time eventually leads to death. This inexorable decline in function, which generally starts by the beginning of one's fourth decade, is universally evident in all physiological processes.

There's Always Hope

We're all aware of those extraordinary athletes who have performed at the top of their sport well beyond normal age expectations. These are the competitors who have pushed the envelope on the performance clock in a remarkable way. People like football's George Blanda, who was thought by Houston to be washed up. After being let go at age 39, he reemerged as a star in Oakland. He played his final game at age 48. Satchel Paige, the first black pitcher in the American League, pitched his last game in 1966. Paige's actual age was always in dispute, but the discovery of his birth certificate in the county health department of Mobile, Alabama, finally confirmed that he was 59 years old when he quit. His autobiography is titled *Maybe I'll Pitch Forever.*

Equally impressive were Gordie Howe, who finally hung up his skates at age 52; Arnold Palmer, who golfed in the 2004 Masters at age 75; and Willie Shoemaker, who at age 54, became the oldest jockey to win the Kentucky Derby (with a little help from his horse Ferdinand). We shouldn't forget, too, Aladàr Gerevich, who holds a record for having won an Olympic gold medal in the same event (fencing) six times. He garnered his last in 1960 when he was 50 years old.

Contemporary tennis fans are awed by Martina Navratilova, who after 18 career singles titles went on to gain further success on the doubles court before retiring at age 49. What fans may not know is that she also coauthored an intriguing 2007 book titled *Art Grand Slam de Paris*, in which she created abstract pieces of art by firing paint-laden tennis balls at a canvas.

The grand title of the world's oldest athlete, however, has to be presented posthumously to John Whittemore, track competitor whose career began at Santa Barbara High School in 1915 and ended in the fall of 2004 when he threw the javelin and discus at the Senior Olympics just before his 105th birthday. At that time, he had established age-group records for the discus, hammer throw, javelin, shot put, and decathlon. During his final competition, he was reported to have remarked, javelin in hand, "If I don't drop it on my foot, I set a world record." Whittemore passed away in April of 2005.

No one knows exactly how long the primary aging process occurs—that is, how long we would live if we could somehow escape the ravages of chronic disease in our older years. But, based on extrapolation of survival curves, it has been suggested that the maximal natural life span of humans could be as high as 120 or 130 years. That's consistent with the oldest recorded human, a French woman named Jeanne Louise Calment who died in 1997 after reaching her 122nd birthday.

Secondary aging refers to a similar deterioration and loss of cellular function that occurs as the aging human is affected by extrinsic factors: disease, malnutrition, and deleterious environmental insults. Myocardial cells fail from the chronic anoxic effect of coronary artery disease. Inadequate levels of exercise and calcium intake lead to bone fractures from osteoporosis. Cigarette smoking may lead to lung cancer.

The progressive rise in longevity in developed nations—doubling in the United States from an average of about 40 years in the mid-1800s to around 80 years at present—is due entirely to a delay in secondary aging. The obvious explanation is the dramatic improvements in health care, sanitation, and nutrition that have occurred over the past 150 years. It is probable, however, that the natural course of primary aging in human beings has not changed over time. We'll discuss this a bit more later on.

Physical Activity and Longevity

It is now well recognized that those who are physically active, on the average, survive longer than those living sedentary lives. The research data clearly indicate that this is specifically an expression of the favorable effect of habitual energy expenditure on secondary aging. Regular exercise reduces health risk factors (dyslipidemia, hypertension, obesity, reduced bone density). In addition, it may have direct protective effects against the atherosclerotic vascular process. Athletes who maintain high levels of sport activity through their adult years can expect to benefit from limited secondary aging.

Whether high levels of physical activity can extend the natural, or primary, aging process is not known, but at present, no evidence supports that idea. The question, of course, would be extraordinarily difficult to address in the experimental setting for human beings. The best we can do is look at animals, who don't live as long and can be coerced to participate as long-term research subjects more easily. Too, in animals, we can expect to more distinctly examine the effects of exercise on the primary aging process.

In a particularly pertinent study (at least for rodents), John Holloszy and Bill Kohrt described the influence of regular running on the longevity of healthy rats who experienced no associated decline in food intake or growth retardation. Beginning at 4 months of age, 62 rats were housed in cages with running wheels. They started out exercising spontaneously an average of 9,173 meters per day. Running distances gradually decreased, falling to 965 meters daily at 34 months of age. Compared with nonexercising control rats, the running rats demonstrated an average life span that was 9% greater (1009 ± 132 days versus 924 days ± 155 days). There was, however, no significant difference between the two groups in maximal duration of life. The age of death of the two oldest rats was 1239 ± 14 days and 1199 ± 44 days in the runners and nonrunners, respectively.

What Factors Delay Primary Aging?

At the present time, only two documented means exist of extending the duration of primary aging—calorie-restricted diets and genetic manipulation. Both of these lines of evidence have been established in animals. As of this moment, their potential application to humans is a tantalizing idea that has not been well explored.

Caloric Restriction

Although the science of aging is generally clouded in mystery, one piece of experimental data has been repeatedly established: In animals, a low-calorie diet that is sufficient in specific nutrients (does not lead to malnutrition) will extend life span. This was first documented in 1917 in rats, and the effect has since been replicated in a wide variety of animals, ranging from fleas to monkeys. The usual experimental technique is to reduce caloric input to about 60% of *ad libitum*, which can be expected to prolong animal life by 25 to 40%. Just how this works is uncertain. Some have suggested that caloric restriction protects mitochondrial function, preserves activity of the electron transport chain, or blocks the deleterious actions of reactive oxygen species. Certain biochemical actions associated with caloric restriction in animals have been observed in humans as well, leading to speculation that *H. sapiens* might similarly benefit from extension of the life span.

Genetic Manipulation

If you happen to be a nematode worm—or are closely related to one—there is hope for you. More than 20 years ago, investigators reported that a single gene mutation in *C. elegans* significantly lengthened the worm's life span, as much as sixfold in some cases. Since that time, antiaging gene mutants have been described in a large number of organisms. The most advanced in terms of evolution is the mouse (with increases that are much more conservative, at 50 to 60%). How these genetic changes act to extend life remains problematic, but it is interesting that most of these gene loci share some connection with alterations in insulin signaling pathways.

It's almost needless to say that the explosive growth in techniques to manipulate gene loci in humans has fueled speculation that someday such fountain-of-youth interventions might extend human life, maybe (gasp!) indefinitely. (This, I believe, should be differentiated from the ideas of Friedrich Nietzsche, who claimed that we will forever relive our lives, just as the time before. The alert reader is, of course, conscious of the similarity of this concept of eternal return to Bill Murray's plight in the film *Groundhog Day*.)

What About Secondary Aging?

We all know that the increase in average life span over the past century is linked to reduced risks of infectious diseases and avoidance of health risk factors such as high-calorie diets, smoking, physical inactivity, and high blood pressure. Dr. Alexander Leaf wanted to look at this more closely. So, he left the safe confines of Massachusetts General Hospital one day and set out to visit remote populations reputed for their longevity in places like Hunza, a kingdom in the Hindu Kush mountains on the China-Afghanistan border; Georgia; and Vilcabamba, in the Andes mountains of Ecuador. (It turned out that the actual longevity of these people was in some doubt. In the latter village, for instance, the oldest citizen was supposedly 134 years old, but turned out at his death to be actually 93.)

Dr. Leaf describes his observations as "a monotonous litany of similar lifestyles."[1] He witnessed the following in all three locations:

- Poor, agrarian culture in which daily hard labor was the norm
- Vigorous daily physical activity beginning in childhood and persisting throughout life
- A vegetarian diet
- Strong support for the elderly

"No one retired or was put on the shelf to feel redundant and useless," he observed. "Chores changed, but the elderly continued to do tasks that, although less vigorous, continued a useful role for them in the community and supported their self-esteem. Old age was greeted with respect rather than derision, and the elders were valued for their wisdom."[1]

Food for thought!

Why Do We Age?

The reason for human aging and its relentless deterioration of physiological function can be sought at two different levels. The first asks for an explanation on an evolutionary basis, seeking an answer in the realm of the order and efficiency of biological processes. The second is mechanistic—just what goes wrong that causes cells, tissues, organs, and entire beings to progressively fail, ultimately extinguishing the life process itself?

Evolutionary Logic of Aging

Scientists are used to—indeed, they usually only feel comfortable—regarding biological processes as satisfying some manner of order, something that makes sense, a function that satisfies a higher benefit for the organism or its social context. Just what that higher order is, of course, is open to all sorts of individual interpretations and topics of debate (Fortunately, for the author, these are not appropriate for these pages.) The generally accepted paradigm for most biologists involves some sense of Darwinian forces, which hold that biological processes should ultimately serve reproductive fitness to maintain survival of the species.

But what good is the aging process? How can it possibly be adaptive? Is aging logical? August Weismann, writing in the early 1900s, proposed that, in fact, this was the case. In a kind of neodarwinism, he suggested that for the survival of populations, older people—who cannot reproduce and drain the resources of a society—are best gotten rid of. Thus, this selective force weeds out unnecessary older persons through the aging process. (One can only hope that Professor Weismann was more fun at dinner parties.)

Well, pretty much no one believes this any more. In fact, most now view the logic of aging in the opposite way: Because older people are past the age of reproduction, they are no longer subject to the controls of natural selection as envisaged by Darwin. Thus, when adverse changes naturally take place in body systems (as outlined in the following section), there is nothing to act (positively or negatively) on these alterations. That is, no force limits functional deterioration.

Mechanisms of Aging

It sometimes seems that the more basic a human function is, the more difficult it is to explain. And, in direct proportion, it engenders more proposed explanations. Why do we sleep? How do we reason? Why do fools fall in love? Who knows? Aging, here, is no exception. Closer looks at genetic, biochemical, and stress determinants of cellular deterioration with time have drawn us closer to new insights, but clear explanations remain elusive. Consequently, proposed mechanisms abound. It has been estimated that more than 300 theories have been put forward for the basis of the aging process, leading Vijg to comment that "there is probably no subspecialty in science in which formulation of theories has been as pervasive as in the science of aging."[2]

You will recall that this chapter starts with an allusion to the role of entropy—a thermodynamic explanation—in the aging process. It sounded good at the time, but now it must be admitted that this only indicates how far behind this author is in his reading. In fact, the last person to truly embrace this idea was Hippocrates, who claimed, 300 years before the birth of Christ, that the aging process reflected a progressive and irreversible loss of heat from the body. (This is only one step above a common idea in the late 1800s that aging was an outcome of intestinal putrefaction.)

One particularly intriguing observation seems to reside over many of the theories about the mechanism of aging. The introduction to this book mentions this briefly: The resting metabolic rate of animals is inversely related to both their body size and their life span. Smaller animals have a higher metabolic rate per kilogram of body mass and a shorter life span than larger ones. Metabolic rate and life span across the animal kingdom generally both relate to body mass$^{0.20}$. That is, all animals turn out to have the same number of metabolic events in their lives, regardless of their size. It's like there is a bank in which a particular number of heartbeats, for instance, are on deposit. All animals, regardless of size, have the same absolute amount in their bank account at birth. The small animals, like mice, make withdrawals rapidly, exhausting their supply and dying in bankruptcy at an earlier age than the big ones, like whales, who withdraw their events over a greater period of time. By this observation, the mechanism for aging must somehow be connected with the rate of metabolic function of the cell.

A number of mechanistic theories for aging are consistent with this concept. In fact, any process that is linked to metabolic rate might fit. So, inevitable adverse DNA mutations within the mitochondria that go unrepaired would work. So would progressive telomere shortening with repetitive cell divisions. Damage from free radicals (reactive oxygen species), altered protein synthesis, or accumulation of metabolic waste (lipofuscin) would be expected to be associated with metabolic activity.

Some have viewed aging as a failure of repair mechanisms to respond to environmentally induced cell damage (heat, ionization, radiation, infection). Others see progressive imbalances in immune function or neuroendocrine regulation as playing a critical role.[2]

Physical Activity
and Body Composition During Aging

Characteristic changes in both body composition and level of habitual physical activity are observed as humans age. Since they can affect physical fitness and its measurement, such factors need to be put into the equation when considering patterns of motor performance associated with senescence.

The hallmark changes in body composition during aging are a progressive loss of lean body mass (skeletal muscle) and an increase in body fat. Percentage of body fat more than doubles between ages 25 and 75, while muscle mass decreases by 3 to 6% per decade. This shift in body composition needs to be taken into account when adjusting physiological variables for body size in studies of aging individuals. Maximal oxygen uptake, for instance, should be expressed relative to lean body mass, not to total body mass (which would provide spuriously lower values as subjects become older).

The course of human aging is also marked by a progressive decline in the level of daily physical activity. Although it is certain that this decline partially reflects the effects of environment, chronic disease, and loss of muscle mass, it has a central biological basis as well. In fact, a progressive decrease in daily energy expenditure (related to body size) is a lifelong feature that begins in early childhood. This phenomenon is observed throughout the animal kingdom and is paralleled by declines in basal metabolic rate and caloric intake. Decreased physical activity in the elderly may adversely accelerate muscle loss and accelerate declines in motor performance while increasing risks for chronic disease.

Difficulties of Studying the Effect
of Aging on Performance

Now we're ready to think about just how the time clock of aging acts to slow motor performance. But first, it's worthwhile to point out the challenges facing investigators who have been trying to answer just this question. The difficulties are many. It's important to keep these in mind as we examine this literature in order to realize how investigators have sought to minimize these obstacles.[3]

Consider, for instance, how you might examine performance on a 1-mile (1.6 km) run during the course of human aging. You could

section, taking a group of 40-, 60-, and 80-year-olds
nifty graph of age versus running times. But that
ork very well because the 80-year-olds are a selective
survived this far and have lost more than a few of
along the way. Too, the three groups might differ in
ctors, such as diet, health, occupation, and habitual
physical activity. And, of course, you'd be comparing three groups of
genetically different people.

A longitudinal study in which you make repeated measurements
of the same subjects as they age makes a lot more sense. But, how
daunting is a 40-year follow-up study? You'll have to keep it funded
for four decades and you can bet on a serious dropout rate. Sadly, it
is likely that many of the subjects will outlive the investigators. The
subjects could alter their lifestyle habits simply because they're in
the study. If the investigators make frequent measurements during
the four decades, there could be a practice effect of performing the
test itself.

A major obstacle to these kinds of aging studies is separating out
the processes of primary and secondary aging. In any longitudinal
study starting with a cohort of 40-year-olds, for example, a certain
number will eventually experience a decrement in performance due
to coronary artery disease (covert or overt), arthritis, or peripheral
vascular disease from diabetes. And each subject will be affected differently (the curve of secondary aging will be unique to each person).

It has been pointed out that assessment of cardiorespiratory function during aging should be conducted by exercise testing, which
discloses limitations of functional reserve that may not be quite so
apparent during rest. Yet the process of performing a cycling or treadmill test in the elderly may itself be influenced by psychological and
noncardiac physiological features that could confound an accurate
assessment of true cardiorespiratory function.

Aging Clock, Motor Capacity, and Athletic Performance

Trained athletes, people who are physically active, and those who
adopt sedentary lifestyles all experience a progressive deterioration
in performance of motor tasks as they reach the elderly adult years.
A great deal of interest surrounds the potential for regular physical
activity and sports participation to counteract this decay of function,

thereby delaying secondary aging and improving the well-being of the elderly. Veteran athletes who continue to participate at highly competitive levels wish to know, as well, by what means training might postpone declines in their performance as they age. As noted previously, the volume of information regarding the role of improved physical activity and sports participation in slowing declines in physical function and performance for the aged has grown tremendously. For the purpose of this short chapter, here are perhaps the four most salient points.

1. *Among the general population, aging is eventually associated with a universal, progressive decline in all forms of motor performance.*[4] The first two decades of life witness a progressive improvement in all types of motor performance. The extent of this rise in physical capabilities is impressive—the average 15-year-old boy can run a mile in almost half the time it takes for a 5-year-old to do it. These dramatic improvements are all pretty much due to increases in body size. That is, children become stronger as they grow, mainly because of muscle enlargement. Improvements in aerobic endurance fitness and exercise economy happen mainly due to increases in leg length and stride frequency. Age-related increases in $\dot{V}O_2$max parallel the larger stroke volumes of bigger heart ventricles. In this age group, then, increases in performance and markers of physiological fitness over time generally reflect the action of hormonal agents that are responsible for promoting body growth.

By the third decade, physical performance measures in healthy, untrained individuals are pretty much at their peak. After this apogee, it all begins to get turned around at age 30. After this, a progressive decline in these same motor measures is observed that persists to the end of the life span. Some of the most commonly reported are outlined in the following list:

- Grip strength
- Dynamic flexor and extensor strength
- Stride length and frequency during locomotion
- Reaction time
- Speed of repetitive movement
- Muscular coordination
- Aiming movements
- Grip precision
- Aerobic endurance performance

- Standing broad jump
- Time of single-foot balance

Although some variation certainly exists, it is generally considered that beyond age 40, the decline of such performance is about 1% per year (10% per decade). It is possible, then, to draw what one might dare to call a lifetime motor performance curve, as in figure 7.1, that would apply to most measures of physical performance measures.

2. *The etiology of decline with aging in any particular form of motor performance rests in deterioration of the anatomical and physiological determinants of that measure.*[5] We've said that the ascending limb of the lifetime motor performance curve is a manifestation of somatic growth (bigger skeletal muscle, heart, lungs). But its descent in the second half of life, quite differently, can be attributed to a universal deterioration of physiological function. The body parts just don't work as well. We need to go no further than the changes in key physiological processes that account for physical performance to see why.

Take maximal oxygen uptake ($\dot{V}O_2max$), for instance. As an indicator of the limits of muscle to utilize oxygen during exercise, $\dot{V}O_2max$ is a critical determinant of performance in aerobic endurance events (running, cycling, swimming). As measured on a maximal treadmill or cycling test, it's a numerical value that reflects the combined function

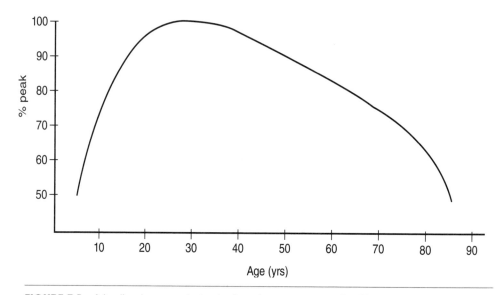

FIGURE 7.1. Idealized curve of physical performance over the lifetime of a human with average physical activity habits. The upward gains in the first half are related principally to somatic growth. After the middle years, performance steadily declines, along with deterioration in physiological function.

of a chain of variables of multiple oxygen delivery and utilization. And all of these factors decline during the aging process.

It is no surprise, then, that $\dot{V}O_2$max falls in the older years. As one might expect, the decline parallels that of aerobic endurance performance (about 10% per decade). All of the physiological determinants of $\dot{V}O_2$max contribute to this change, including declines in maximal heart rate, stroke volume, arterial-venous oxygen difference, muscle capillarization, muscle oxidative capacity (mitochondrial density), and blood flow to muscles. Other features share in the age-related decline of cardiorespiratory function during exercise. The heart muscles' ability to contract and relax are compromised, arterial blood pressure rises, the arteries become stiffer, the enzyme content and cell metabolic efficiency declines, and the function of the lungs decreases. It's not a pretty picture.

Declines in muscle strength in the elderly can be attributed to a progressive loss of skeletal muscle mass, or *sarcopenia*, which in turn reflects decreases in both cross-sectional area and number of fibers. Here, there is also some contribution of both shrinking size and declining function. This process of muscle atrophy, which is most obvious in fast-twitch (Type II) fibers, causes a decrease in the size of the muscles which amounts to—here's that number again—10% per decade. That means that by age 80, the typical person has lost 40% of the muscle mass he had in his prime at age 40.

Neurological degeneration adds to the decline in muscle strength with aging. The motor nerve cells that are responsible for activating muscle fibers are lost at the now predictable rate of 1% yearly. Similar loss of neurons in the central nervous system explains deterioration of reaction times and motor coordination.

Such decays in performance-related physiologies are, in turn, manifestations of some combination of those 300 possible aging mechanisms we talked about before. Certain of these are probably more likely candidates: low-grade inflammation with damaging effects of circulating cytokines, mitochondrial aging (mutations and deletions, diminished protein synthesis), uncoupling of excitation and contraction caused by denervation, nuclear apoptosis, and accumulated oxidative stress.

It has not been lost on those who care about such things that the features of physiological decline of aging closely resemble those observed when subjects adopt a sedentary lifestyle or are forced into prolonged periods of bed rest. Given the significant decline in daily energy expenditure with aging, then, reductions in habitual activity might be expected to contribute to falls in physiological and motor performance. Just how much, though, remains uncertain. Studies comparing the decline of $\dot{V}O_2$max with age in athletes with that of sedentary subjects suggest that physical inactivity itself might account for as much as 50% of physiological decline. And, of course, we could argue that the arrow can go in the other direction: Loss of physical fitness might cause the elderly to reduce their levels of physical activity. In any event, it's a circular effect that calls for an argument to keep elderly persons physically active.

3. *The anatomical and physiological effects of exercise training directly counter those of the aging process.*[6] Reflecting on this statement, you can't help but be struck with a rather remarkable idea. The beneficial effects of regular exercise, of physical training, are just those that would be expected to counter this deterioration in function that occurs with aging. If an elderly person keeps physically active, wouldn't that delay the aging process? We know that regular aerobic endurance exercise increases $\dot{V}O_2$max and improves the heart's pumping capacity, develops growth of muscle capillaries, and stimulates the metabolic machinery in the mitochondria. Resistance training augments strength, fiber size, and neurological activation of our skeletal muscles. These are, in fact, just those items on the list of deterioration we see with senescence. In exercise, then, we should have a powerful antiaging agent. If not a fountain of youth, at least a very useful way of reducing and delaying the functional deterioration of getting old. This would be true, that is, if the responses of the body to exercise training are the same for the 65-year-old retiree as for the 22-year-old cross country runner. Is this so?

No person has probably thought about this more than Bill Evans. In the 1980s, when he was the head of the physiology lab at the Human Nutrition Research Center on Aging at Tufts University, he set out to answer that question. Professor Evans noted that past research on exercise efforts in aged persons had simply been based on animal studies and extrapolations from results of younger subjects. This didn't make much sense. His idea was to take elderly subjects themselves, put them in the testing laboratory, submit them to exercise training programs, and see what happened.

He and his colleagues started by looking at the effects of periods of weight training. They went out to a local nursing home and found 87- to 96-year-old women who would be willing to break away from their TV sets and perform a prescribed regular resistance program for 8 weeks. The results? Their average muscle strength tripled and their muscle size increased by 10%. Then came a 12-week strength training program in 60- to 70-year-old men that resulted in a mean increase in their lifting ability from 44 to 85 pounds (20 to 40 kg). Subsequent studies found the same thing. So, there you have it. Good evidence has it that elderly persons are just as capable of increasing muscle strength with regular weight training as younger ones.

The same thing is observed with aerobic endurance training. If you put sexagenarians into a regular walking or running program, their maximal oxygen uptake increases by 20 to 30%. You'll also see the same magnitude of increases in muscle oxidative capacity that young adults experience under the same regimen. Concluded Evans, "Advanced age is not a static, irreversible biological condition of unwavering decreptitude. Rather, it's a dynamic state that, in most people, can be changed for the better no matter how many years they've lived or neglected their body in the past."[6]

Think about that for a moment. If a program of aerobic endurance or resistance training can improve function in the elderly by even 30%, that's the same thing as reversing the aging process by roughly three decades. Here's a way in which one can truly make the clock of physiological time move backward.

I once heard Bill Evans deliver a presentation on this, his favorite subject at a sports medicine meeting up in Lake Placid. And, you know, by the end, his findings were just so persuasive that I suspect half the audience was thinking that they just couldn't wait to get old. His slides of smiling 90-year-old people lifting weights are memorable. Along with his coworker Irwin Rosenberg, Evans went on to publish a book called *Biomarkers*, which imparts not only enthusiasm but also practical exercise advice for the elderly. It's a classic. Why this is not included in the "Medicare and You" information packet one receives from the government at age 65 is a mystery to me.

So, when you get to that age "when you get winded playing chess, when you're still chasing women but can't remember why, when you stoop down to tie your shoelaces and ask yourself, 'What else can I do while I'm down here?'"[7] don't forget Evans' advice. "The markers of biological aging can be more than altered: In the case of specific physiological functions, they can actually be reversed."[6]

4. *Veteran athletes who continue training exhibit superior fitness in the elderly years compared to nonathletes. The rate of decline of physiological performance, however, is similar in the two groups.*[8] What does all this mean for senior athletes? Will continued sports training prevent the functional declines that come with aging? Specifically, as David Proctor and Michael Joyner posed the question "Exercise and aging: Can the biological clock be stopped?" The answer is probably not. The senior athlete demonstrates superior physical fitness and physiological capacities compared to the nonathletic elderly person. This gap will be maintained as long as the athlete continues training. But the rate of decay in these features over time appears to be the same, whether you're a superb master athlete or not.

In addressing this question, the most frequent variable studied has been $\dot{V}O_2$max. Values of $\dot{V}O_2$max in highly trained male aerobic endurance athletes aged 60 to 70 are often around 50 to 60 ml/kg/min, or almost double that of their sedentary peers. $\dot{V}O_2$max is lower for females than for males, but the magnitude of differences between the elderly trained and sedentary are similar.

Some early studies indicated that this superior level of aerobic fitness would also delay the decline of $\dot{V}O_2$max over time by as much as 50% of that of nonathletes. However, two subsequent meta-analyses of multiple studies that provided a broader assessment—one in men, the other in women—have failed to bear out this optimism. Margaret Fitzgerald and colleagues reviewed data on the decline of $\dot{V}O_2$max with aging from 109 cross-sectional studies in female subjects. The women were divided into three groups: those who were training in aerobic endurance, active, and sedentary. The rate of decline of $\dot{V}O_2$max with age was found to be directly related to exercise status, with decreases of 6.2, 4.4, and 3.5 ml/kg/min per decade in the three groups, respectively (figure 7.2a). However, no differences in reduction rate of aerobic fitness were found between groups when values were expressed as percentage change from $\dot{V}O_2$max at age 25 (losses of 10.0-10.9% per decade).

A similar metaanalysis of 242 studies in males by Teresa Wilson and Hirofumi Tanaka revealed similar findings. (It is not surprising that training mileage in the endurance runners decreased in direct proportion to age, but it is rather astonishing to note that they were still putting in an average of 50 kilometers a week at age 65.) Rates of both absolute declines in $\dot{V}O_2$max with age and percentage change from age 25 were not significantly different among the three groups (figure 7.2b). These authors concluded that "the age-related rate of decline in $\dot{V}O_2$max is not associated with habitual exercise status in healthy men."[8] And the same appears to be true in women as well.

Patterns of decline in different forms of athletic performance have typically been examined by plotting graphs of age-related world records or performances in certain championship events. This approach, of course, suffers from several of the methodological problems outlined earlier in this chapter. Most particularly, in almost

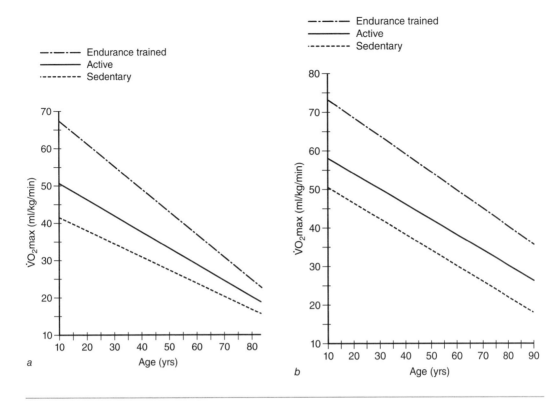

FIGURE 7.2. Meta-analyses of changes in V̇O₂max with aging. *(a)* In women, rate of decrease was greatest for those who were aerobic endurance trained and was lowest for sedentary subjects. *(b)* In men, no differences in rate of decline in aerobic fitness were observed between trained, normally active, and sedentary groups.

(a) Reprinted from M.D. Fitzgerald et al., 1997, "Age-related declines in maximal aerobic capacity in regularly exercising vs. sedentary women: a meta-analysis," *Journal of Applied Physiology* 83: 160-165. Used with permission.

(b) Reprinted from T.M. Wilson and H. Tanaka, 2000, "Meta-analysis of the age-associated decline in maximal aerobic capacity in men: relation to training status," *American Journal of Physiology: Heart and Circulation* 278: H829-H834. Used with permission.

all cases, there is no means by which comparisons can be made with changes in performance of nonathletes. But these graphs do give us some general insights on what happens to highly trained seniors as they age.

Fall off in 10K race times typically begins around age 35, with a steady decline until the late 50s, and then more precipitous decline after that. An examination of world-record holders at the U.S. Masters National Championships in 2002 demonstrates a 40% decrement in velocity in the 100-meter, 800-meter, and 10K running events between ages 35 and 75. This is pretty much what Hirofumi Tanaka and Doug Seals found when they plotted world-record times and top freestyle performances in the U.S. masters swimming championships from 1991 to 1995. Between age 40 and 70, the decrement in 1.5K times was approximately 44%, or about 15% per decade. Declines in men and women were about the same until age 80, when females dropped off more.

Same thing for cyclists. Records from the 2002 U.S. Cycling Federation 20K races show a 30% decline between age 40 and 80. The difference in age-group first-place finish times for the 40-year-olds and 70-year-olds in the Masters National Rowing Regatta in 2000 was approximately 26%. In these aerobic endurance sports, then, the rates of decline in performance are similar (10% per decade). They generally match those of physiological markers ($\dot{V}O_2$max), which, as we've seen, are comparable in athletes and nonathletes.

The same performance decline of 10% per decade is described in national records of weightlifting and powerlifting. From these data, Professors Proctor and Joyner concluded that "the average rates of change for weightlifting records, as a function of age, are not much less than the rates of strength loss in the general sedentary population. However, strength-trained athletes are stronger and more powerful at any given age, providing higher functional reserve."[8]

This statement seems to pretty much sum up, based on current data, our understanding of how aging affects elite-level veteran athletes. Their performance is superior—and will continue to be as long as training is maintained—but the disappointing effects of the aging process take the same toll.

Notes

1. Leaf, A. 1988. "The aging process: Lessons from observations in man." *Nutrition Review* 46: 40-44.

2. Read more about what makes us age in the following sources: Austad, S.N. 1998. "Theories of aging: An overview." *Aging* 10: 146-147. Hepple, R.T. 2009. "Why eating less keeps mitochondria working in aged skeletal muscle." *Exercise Sport Science Review* 37: 23-28. Van Remmen, H., M.L. Hamilton, and A. Richardson. 2003. "Oxidative damage to DNA and aging." *Exercise Sport Science Review* 31: 149-153. Vijg, J. 2007. *Aging of the genome. The dual role of DNA in life and death*. Oxford: Oxford University Press.

3. The difficulties in figuring out how aging affects physical performance are described in detail here: Groeller, H. 2008. "The physiology of aging in active and sedentary humans." In *Physiological bases of human performance during work and exercise*, ed. N.A.S. Taylor and H. Groeller, 289-306. Philadelphia: Elsevier.

4. See the following articles: Spiroduso, W.W., K.L. Francis, and P.G. Mac Rae. 2005. *Physical dimensions of aging*. 2nd ed. Champaign, IL: Human Kinetics. Stones, M.J., and A. Kozma. 1985. "Physical performance." In *Aging and human performance*, ed. N. Charness, 261-292. London: Wiley.

5. For further reading: Tanaka, H., and D.R. Seals. 2008. "Endurance exercise performance in Masters athletes: Age-associated changes and underlying mechanisms." *Journal of Physiology* 586: 55-63.

6. See the following: Evans, W., and I.H. Rosenberg. 1991. *Biomarkers*. New York: Simon and Schuster. Rogers, M.A., and W.J. Evans. 1993. "Changes in skeletal muscle with aging: Effects of exercise training." *Exercise Sport Science Review* 21: 65-102.

7. Burns, George. 1983. *How to live to be one hundred or more*. New York: G.P. Putnam's Sons.

8. More information on the effects of training by veteran athletes can be found in the following articles: Fitzgerald, M.D., H. Tanaka, Z.V. Tran, and D.R. Seals. 1997. "Age-related declines in maximal aerobic capacity in regularly exercising vs. sedentary women: A meta-analysis." *Journal of Applied Physiology* 83: 160-165. Proctor, D.N., and M.J. Joyner. 2008. "Exercise and aging: Can the biological clock be stopped?" In *Physiological bases of human performance during work and exercise*, ed. N.A.S. Taylor and H. Groeller, 313-319. Philadelphia: Elsevier. Wilson, T.M., and H. Tanaka. 2000. "Meta-analysis of the age-associated decline in maximal aerobic capacity in men: Relation to training status." *American Journal of Physiology* 278: H829-H834.

TAKE-HOME MESSAGES

1. Beyond age 40, all athletes, despite highly intensive training regimens, inevitably experience a progressive fall in performance. This decline largely reflects anatomical and physiological deterioration that is part of the body's general aging process. Changes in other determinants, such as body composition, physical activity, and training volume, also contribute.

2. Continued training in the elderly years will keep the athlete's performance superior to that of nonathletes.

3. Persistent training will not, however, lessen the rate of fall in performance, which is similar (a loss of about 10% per decade) to that of those who don't train.

4. These patterns are evident in all forms of sport and are not dramatically different in males and females.

CODA

It's time to sum up. We've seen that the essence of sport competition—testing the outer limits of our muscle machinery to endure, generate power, or finely tune visual-motor events—is intimately connected with the ticking of our internal clocks. And not just one, but many. The mechanisms of these time pieces, crafted by eons of biological evolution, were originally designed for survival. In sport, of course, their meaning has been transformed. For sure, they create personal challenges and fulfillment for the fortunate athletes among us. But, as well, they've become a core element of our contemporary culture, all the way from providing vicarious pleasure to those of us watching TV to creating identities for our countries and educational institutions.

We've observed that time may be on our side, but when our biological clocks govern motor performance, they often do so at a subconscious level. Still, it is evident that successful athletes can cognitively manipulate the dictates of their clocks through training and competition strategies that can improve sport performance.

So, what better way to summarize than to rewind a personal time machine to the 1965 Rose Bowl game? (That's got to be *clock 1*, the one that defines the rise and fall of our physical abilities over the course of a lifetime.) The University of Michigan Wolverines versus the Beavers of Oregon State. It's 75 degrees F with the San Gabriel Mountains as the backdrop. This sure beats New Year's Day in Ann Arbor. You'll find me in section 15, row 10, seat 14. From there, the ticking of all these clocks is, indeed, quite tumultuous.

It's third down and five at midfield. Quarterback Bob Timberlake breaks the huddle, glances up at the scoreboard. *Clock 2* says 2:14 to play. End John Henderson is split out wide to the right. Snap of the ball. *Clock 3*. The central pattern generator in Henderson's spinal cord fires the sequential contractions of his leg muscles, driving him down the field. Post pattern. *Clock 4*. In the brain stem. Turning up the tempo of the spinal cord oscillator. Faster! Faster! *Clock 5*. The circadian timepiece in the Michigan end's suprachiasmatic nucleus has tuned itself to a top performance in the late afternoon. *Clock 6*. His pineal gland is telling the SCN that now is the time. Went right by that defender! He's all alone, out in the open. Timberlake fires a perfect spiral. *Clock 7.* In the basal ganglia. Watching. Timing. The ball floating in slow motion. Henderson can see the laces. Arms out for the catch. *Clock 8.* A flag lies on the turf. Fans, it's coming back. The 25-second clock had expired. The Wolverines are penalized 5 yards for delay of game. (No matter. Final score: Michigan 34, Oregon State 7.)

INDEX

Note: The italicized *f and t* following page numbers refer to figures and tables,

Thomas W. Rowland, MD, is a pediatric cardiologist at the Baystate Medical Center in Springfield, Massachusetts, where he established an exercise testing laboratory. The author of *Children's Exercise Physiology, Second Edition*, and editor of the journal *Pediatric Exercise Science,* he has extensive research experience in exercise physiology of children.

Dr. Rowland has served as president of the North American Society for Pediatric Exercise Medicine (NASPEM) and was on the board of trustees of the American College of Sports Medicine (ACSM). He is past president of the New England chapter of the ACSM and received the Honor Award from that organization in 1993.

After receiving his BS and MD degrees from the University of Michigan in 1965 and 1969, Dr. Rowland completed postgraduate training at the University of Colorado and Boston Children's Hospital. He is professor of pediatrics at Tufts University School of Medicine and a past adjunct professor of exercise science at the University of Massachusetts.

Dr. Rowland is a competitive tennis player and distance runner. He and his wife, Margot, reside in Longmeadow, Massachusetts.

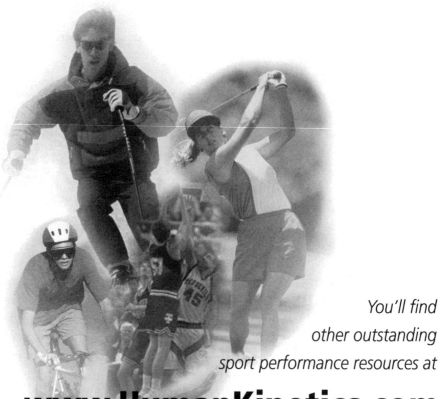

*You'll find
other outstanding
sport performance resources at*

www.HumanKinetics.com

In the U.S. call

1-800-747-4457

Australia.............................. 08 8372 0999
Canada 1-800-465-7301
Europe..................... +44 (0) 113 255 5665
New Zealand........................ 0800 222 062